Body
Esteem

Body Esteem

Piece of Cake & Peace of Mind

Be Your Own Kind of
Beautiful

Susan Walker, M.S., L.P.C.

Contents

Introduction
Body Esteem

"Beauty begins the moment you decide to be yourself."
—Coco Chanel

My husband and I have birthdays one day apart, and we love to travel and give one another gifts that create a memory! One year his gift was to jump out of an airplane, and I elected to play it safe and have a Swedish massage. I consider myself somewhat of a connoisseur since a great massage recharges my batteries and helps me relax and unwind. Much to my surprise my masseuse was blind and told me that if she did not drape my body properly not to worry because she could not see. It was the best massage I have ever had, and I was especially impressed with her optimism about life. She played the violin, read mystery novels, travels, and has a family and career. However, something she told me was very interesting. She said, "People are so self-conscious about their body that they are often relieved when they discover I am blind." She went on to tell me that they have a sense of freedom knowing that she cannot "see" them in the traditional sense.

This enlightening experience reaffirmed what I have observed in my clinical practice of more than twenty-five years where every day, I help people with their body image issues. I have realized from many years of clinical experience that body esteem is more essential now than ever before. The definition of body esteem is the level and degree of positiveness that an individual clearly attributes to his or her own body. It is also the significance that one gives to the different parts (e.g., breasts, stomach, hips, or thighs) of the body and to the appearance of these body parts. In essence, when one learns to give more value to each body part and to their entire body, they succeed in enhancing their body esteem. Self-esteem and body esteem are highly correlated, and the higher your self-esteem, the more likely you are to have better body esteem.

My hope is that I can impart some of my clinical knowledge and make a difference in how you view your body. Your body is already beautiful. I can feel you shaking your head, and you may be in disagreement and feel compelled to tell me you wish to make changes with your body. My message is that you may or may not choose to improve your body, but taking responsibility for your mental and physical health is paramount for prevention and wellness. Assigning a more positive value to your body will bring you peace of mind. Beautiful body esteem can be achieved by all, and this book will reframe and redefine your body image. Selfies, swimsuit season, shopping, and intimacy with your partner all become more pleasurable when you are confident and enjoy your physical presence.

Similarly, you can experience an ease about your physical appearance when you do not allow societal norms and a specific standard of beauty dictate how your feel about yourself. You will discover body enrichment techniques that build better body image. I invite you to leave behind not wanting to be seen in a picture, avoiding the mirror, socially isolating yourself, or not engaging in physical affection from hugs to kisses to sex. All of these feelings of discomfort and distress dissipate as you improve your body esteem. You will discover how emotional and physical well-being bring satisfaction and joy to your life.

Let's reflect on the history and evolution of why positive body image is relevant. Body image was initially defined as a person's perception of the aesthetics or sexual attractiveness of their own body. The phrase *body image* was first coined by the Austrian neurologist and psychoanalyst Paul Schilder in his book *The Image and Appearance of Human Body* in 1935. Notice that timing—at the dawn of Hollywood and cameras—although, the emphasis of placing great value on the human body has been around forever. Pierre-Auguste Renoir was a French artist who was a leading painter in the development of the Impressionist style and was a celebrator of beauty and feminine sensuality. The voluptuous bathing beauties that he painted have certainly stood the test of time and were revered among other Impressionist artists such as Claude Monet. But portraits and paintings were extremely expensive and often left to the interpretation of the artist. The emergence of the camera was a game changer regarding how we started to think about ourselves and how we look to others.

Beauty and the Beast

The musical and movie *Beauty and the Beast* serves as a reminder that we can find attractiveness in all aspects such as our personality (e.g., compassion or sense of humor), physical appearance (e.g., freckles or dimples), and intelligence (e.g., knowledge acquired as a seasoned traveler or avid reader). The societal pressures and expectation of beauty and body image are more prevalent today than ever before with social media. The concept of body image extends over a number of disciplines including psychology, medicine, philosophy, and cultural and feminist studies. The term has become commonplace throughout our vernacular as a type of shorthand for how one is to "look" based on societal norms. But the pressure to present and express ourselves physically has risen to a whole new level on social media, which may apply more pressure to be thin or set the standard for a specific image that one should acquire. It also adds immediate feedback regarding style such as "live from the red carpet" and a certain nationally televised lingerie fashion show. Across these disciplines and media there is no consensus definition. A person's body image is thought to be, in part, a product of their personal experiences, personality, and various social and cultural forces.

Over the years I have had the pleasure of working with ballerinas, gymnasts, and ice skaters, all who are subjected to strict standards due to the fact that the competition and/or coaches often impose a particular body weight, and the competition itself requires precision for scoring and esthetics. Misty Copeland, a ballerina for the American Ballet Theatre, joined the company at age nineteen when she was 5'2" and weighed 108 pounds. She began bingeing on a box of Krispy Kreme doughnuts with a glass of wine while watching episodes of *Sex and the City*. She suffered an injury and was put on birth control pills to jumpstart her menstrual cycle, and she gained weight, as many young women do when taking hormone replacement therapy. She was summoned by the "artistic staff" and was told that her body had changed. "The lines you're creating don't look the way they used to. We'd like to see you lengthen." This seems to be code in the ballerina world for you have gained weight, and you need to lose it.

Over time she made peace with her body and became the first African American dancer to perform a featured solo in two decades. She was headlining in the ballet *Firebird*. When she saw a billboard on the Metropolitan Opera House featuring her wearing a red leotard, with her chest and back arched, her full, feminine breasts and round butt prominent, she began to sob and thought that she looked so entirely different than what people expect in a ballerina. In her memoir she writes about her reaction identifying, "beauty, power—it was a woman, and it was me!"

She has successfully celebrated her lovely feminine body that defies the standard or paradigm for ballerinas. Today, women of all ages everywhere are waking up to their own physical power whereby we are no longer willing to self-impose physical perfection. Like Misty Copeland, we're beginning to look at ourselves through our own lens instead of through the eyes of others. In order to change the standard and paradigm of how we view our bodies, we have to become more acquainted and knowledgeable about our body intelligence.

We often acquire knowledge on how to improve our brain health, emotional intelligence, and mindset, but equally important are methods on how to improve our body esteem. Body esteem encompasses a full spectrum, and regardless of where you fall on that spectrum, there may or may not be room for improvement. Through my clinical experience I have developed what I refer to as a body esteem quotient (BEQ), which means that one can increase their knowledge and understanding on how to acquire body esteem. There are four quotients that comprise body esteem quotient (BEQ): psychological quotient (PQ), nutritional quotient (NQ), exercise quotient (EQ), and fashion quotient (FQ). Throughout this book, I will introduce you to the concepts that make up these quotients and present you with tips, tools, and techniques that will help you to master all four quotients, which in turn will improve your overall body esteem quotient (BEQ).

My husband and I own Walker Wellness Clinic, and our primary headquarters are on the campus of Cooper Aerobics Center in Dallas, Texas. As a psychotherapist and clinical director, I have acquired a wealth of knowledge on preventive medicine, wellness research, and mental health. We also have a location in Houston, Texas. In both locations, we work with body image issues, disordered eating, and formal eating disorders. Our understanding of how we optimize our psychological and physical health has grown exponentially. The possibilities are endless: improve your brain health via exercise and music, set boundaries in regards to the negative influence that social media or others may have over your body image, complete an annual preventive physical exam to maintain wellness, improve your mental health via psychological assessments, participate in biofeedback to manage your stress, and incorporate methods from this book to increase your body esteem quotient (BEQ). While it would be wonderful to meet with you in person, I have written this book to share with you what I have learned over years of clinical practice in working with experts in the field. The tools and techniques here have been modified to help us all come to terms with how we think about our bodies and to finally embrace every glorious, unique, and appealing feature of what embodies our spirits!

There She Is, Miss America

Throughout my clinical experience, I have seen that there may be a tendency to overestimate or underestimate one's body size. A person's perception of their appearance can be different from how others actually perceive them. I'm sure you've had a moment when you listened to a recording of your voice and were surprised that it sounded so different from how you hear your own voice. The same can be true of how we each perceive our own body. Some may see their body image as distorted and do not have an accurate depiction of their body composition. I'll teach you how to learn to trust your personal judgement when it comes to assessing your body size and weight. Often, we perceive our physical appearance in relation to others or in comparison to some cultural idea, and this leads to unhealthy body image. It is analogous to being colorblind, but as you improve your body esteem quotient (BEQ), you will have an accurate assessment of just how wonderful your body is and can be.

There was a lot of news coverage when the Miss America pageant announced that contestants would no longer participate in the swimsuit competition. I think it is time for all of us to set aside our own "competition" over our various body parts and how we look as a whole. If you are comparing your body to Miss America pageant contestants—or anyone else for that matter—this may lead to poor body image. However, I have confidence in your ability to overcome this comparative analysis and enjoy each person for their own beauty without comparing yourself or letting it affect your body image.

The incongruities between societal norms and expectations may create confusion and disappointment, but I am confident you will eventually experience body empowerment. Your inner dialogue (i.e., I wish I had a body like Nicole Kidman because she looks like a goddess!) will diminish once you no longer impose unrealistic expectations onto your body. In a group therapy session, I brought in pictures of celebrities without makeup and without any digital filters or enhancements. Interestingly, none of the patients were able to identify them, and all reported no desire to emulate these women. This book will teach each of us to readjust the paradigm of desired physical perfection!

The Catwalk

I have always had a passion for fashion! I have had the honor and privilege to chair many fashion shows and charity luncheons, but one of my favorites was for the Dallas Symphony Orchestra League called "Springtime in Paris." I am an advocate for raising money for young and talented musicians! I used the members of the charity as fashion models, retailers provided their clothing, and a local jewelry store draped them in diamonds. The member models were holding musical instruments (e.g., clarinet and flute) on the catwalk with music from French composers playing in the background as each strutted down the runway. My goal was to raise as much money as possible by selling the clothing, jewelry, and hydrangea centerpieces and conserve cost by not hiring professional models. Our lovely participants and my philosophy to be your own kind of beautiful showed us all that while none of us have the same body, we are all beautiful in our own way. The audience cheered for the ladies and loved it!

As an essential piece of media through advertising, it appears that our culture has encouraged many unhealthy role models with the capturing of the "most attractive" of us in the modeling business. Across the globe, we are beginning to see a wider representation of women and bodies that is literally changing the shape of modeling. The strong movement by women today who want to take charge of their own body image, has been put into action. France now requires medical clearance for models to protect their health and to prevent formal eating disorders.

Other countries such as India, Israel, Italy, and Spain are following suit and implementing ways to promote the well-being of models. The Council of Fashion Designers of America now has guidelines for its members. Perhaps these changes in an industry that has long set the standard for "beauty" may now serve as an opportunity to take back our own power and reject any pre-set idea of how we are supposed to look.

And the Oscar Goes To . . .

We all seem to be enchanted by Hollywood. Of course, enchantment is their business! But when we begin to compare ourselves to the high bar of Hollywood, we're setting ourselves up for disappointment. Even the actresses and actors in the business of Hollywood feel the pressure of great value being placed on their physical appearance. And that often cascades over to the rest of us, particularly in our pursuit of becoming thinner. However, more celebrities, such as Scarlet Johansson, are speaking out as she did when asked about a report of losing fourteen pounds for a movie role. She stated, "I'm a petite person to begin with, so the idea of losing this amount of weight is utter lunacy. If I were to lose fourteen pounds, I'd have to part with both arms. And a foot. I'm frustrated with the irresponsibility of the tabloid media who sell the public ideas about what we should look like and how we should get there." Other actresses and celebrities are also redefining the standard of beauty and how they refuse to succumb to this societal expectation.

Am I suggesting that you not watch movies or have an Oscar party? Absolutely not, but be cognizant of the influence that the media has over you. This phenomenon dates back for decades since we have been enthralled with icons from James Bond to Lady Gaga. All of these characters and the actors and actresses who play them served as an embodiment of fantasies of masculine or feminine beauty to which movie goers aspire to emulate. A great film allows you to escape into fantasy and can be very alluring. However, it can become problematic when one blurs the lines between an illusion and reality. Resist comparing your body to unattainable expectations, which lead to becoming self-critical of your own body. It is possible to learn to appreciate others' aesthetics and physical appearance without desiring to look like them.

I am not referring to changing your hairstyle or color to match that of Jessica Chastain. One caveat is if you are looking for a quick fix or to mimic other's appearance, the aforementioned may become a slippery slope and lead to obsessionality. I would encourage you to pursue your unique hairstyle and color that compliment your face and complexion. Others are altering perceived imperfections, and some are attempting to acquire features admired in others. Cosmetic surgeons commonly report their patient's use of celebrity names to describe their desired physical attribute (i.e., a butt like Kim Kardashian or lips like Angelina Jolie). While we are aware of the influence that Hollywood plays in our desire to look more like those adored, we have to accept responsibility and safeguard ourselves on how we allow this to affect us. The media has a profound effect on all ages and especially children and adolescents, who face an unrelenting barrage of media imagery daily. We can teach our children and ourselves to limit excessive exposure to media and build body esteem.

Picture Perfect

Seeking perfection for your body is stressful, but aspiring to be your very best is attainable. Pursuing the perfect body is one of the reasons that many of us may experience feelings of inadequacies. Perfectionism is a personality trait that is genetically predisposed. It is quite common among highly intelligent people, and it serves them well for the most part. However, if perfectionism is taken to the extreme with your body image, it can be self-punitive. You may become rigid and inflexible with your food intake and feel guilty if you do not exercise every day because you fear losing control and feeling powerless. Achievement-oriented people are proactive and productive, but simply reframe a more realistic and optimistic approach when it comes to body empowerment.

More often than not, it appears that perfectionists feel the need to be validated and accepted by others, and they want to please others at the risk of not pleasing themselves. When your partner makes comments about another body, you internalize it and think it is indirectly pointed at you. If you are an approval seeker, you may not experience the happiness that you deserve because you need that stamp of approval from those around you. This extends to how you feel about your body, and often not just your body as a whole, but each individual feature. I often see people, especially women, who are fit and have beautiful features and still focus on every perceived imperfection rather than celebrating and enjoying their body. The Time's Up movement has gained force and momentum in terms of what we are no longer willing to tolerate when it comes to how others treat us, and how we treat ourselves. The time is now for us to move to peace and enjoyment of how we look and who we are. The drive for perfection leads to distorted thinking, which creates a fracture in how we care for our bodies. Perfectionism may not manifest itself in all aspects of one's life but often is seen in body image issues.

You may have fears about losing control and letting go of perfectionism as it relates to your body. Perhaps you are afraid that you will let yourself go and no longer care about your appearance or body. The process of gaining control over other areas in your life where you may feel powerless allows you to no longer self-impose perfectionism. If you have experienced some life-changing events that are stressful, such as divorce or career changes, you may have felt that you no longer have control over your life. One of my favorite quotes is by an unknown author: "We can't always choose the music life plays for us, but we can choose how we dance to it." I encourage you to identify what control you do have over your life, and in turn you will not be as self-critical when it comes to your body. There is a strong correlation between feeling powerless over your circumstances and controlling your food intake, exercise routine, and how you see yourself.

Moreover, gaining more knowledge in regard to your body intelligence is powerful and will help you differentiate between empirically researched literature in this book and nonscientific information that may not be valid or reliable. As you acquire more knowledge based on the most current research about the four quotients, you will diminish your obsessionality regarding your body. You will no longer obsess over your weight, calories, and clothing sizes, and compare yourself to others; instead, you will actually feel empowered because you will no longer fall prey to the propaganda and projected 70 billion weight loss industry in 2018. You will be able to have your cake and eat it too because you deserve a piece of cake and peace of mind!

Four Factors of Body Esteem: Psychology, Nutrition, Exercise, and Fashion

My mother once said to me that my life experiences and clinical knowledge on a subject matter that is critically important could potentially educate others to have better body image from an early age. Why have I chosen to write this book now? The timing is critical in the age of social media, body bullying, and the desire to implement change. My battle cry is that you embrace the philosophy "Be Your Own Kind of Beautiful." My hope is that you will be kinder to yourself and establish more autonomy. My gift to you is to help you build better body esteem and experience a better quality of life.

This book will introduce you to a new way to think about your body through a psychological quotient (PQ), nutrition quotient (NQ), exercise quotient (EQ), and fashion quotient (FQ) that foster body esteem and improve your overall body esteem quotient (BEQ). Clearly, all of these factors are important aspects of learning to flatter your figure and enhance your body image. In my clinical experience, all of these variables go hand and hand, and one of them cannot stand alone as a component of your body esteem quotient. It is my hope to revolutionize how one sees themselves when they look in the mirror and to embrace the concept of not only learning to accept our bodies but making them the very best they can possibly be.

Chapter 1
What Are You Weighting For?

*"Make your life a masterpiece; imagine no
limitations on what you can be, have, or do."*
—Brian Tracy

Prince William and Kate, Duchess of Cambridge, first met while studying at St. Andrews University in Scotland. Kate was the shy, sporty, history of art major who caught Prince William's eye when she was on the catwalk in the university fashion show. Prince William was a world-famous prince who won over Kate's heart with his wit, charm, and kindness. They dated for almost ten years before they became the royal couple. By this time the duchess was nicknamed "Waity Katie," as Prince William had not popped the question to his long-time girlfriend. We will forever have memories etched in our minds of the royal wedding and when the couple wowed the crowd with the infamous kiss. Today they are now one of the most photographed couples in the world, and their love story is one for the history books, as fairytales really can come true! I would say that some things are worth waiting for, and perhaps sometimes we wait too long. What are you waiting (weighting) for?

Imagine you are at a fountain in the midst of lovely gardens and you are tossing coins and making a wish for something. What would you wish for—a better body, a new relationship, erasure of the pain and suffering of losing a loved one, a new career, to look like someone else, or possibly a new life? What are you waiting (weighting) for? Perhaps you are waiting to start dating when you lose weight, grieve the loss of your broken engagement, have the perfect body, or fit into a size 8? What about cultivating a better quality of life now where you are motivated to reach for the stars and make all of your dreams come true?

When you have hope for the future and can visualize the changes you want to make, the likelihood of reaching your goals becomes much more achievable. For years, psychologists have known that if a patient is hopeful about their progress in psychotherapy, that the patient can make steady progress, even given setbacks. If you have lost hope or confidence in your abilities to succeed, I am an optimistic realist, and I believe that you can make the changes you envision. My clinical skills have served my patients well, and I am here to help you so you can stop the waiting game.

Motivation is a necessary component that empowers you to accomplish your dreams, hopes, and aspirations. Imagine waking up in the morning and having the passion to accomplish your goals because you have a clear sense of purpose in doing so. Motivation is a correlation of cognitions and behaviors that are in sync with one another so that you can have maximum performance. It is analogous to a symphony or band where all of the instruments have been finely tuned, backed by many well-rehearsed sessions, and the orchestration comes together to make magnificent music! In my clinical opinion people are highly motivated due to their ability to take strategic risks, build self-esteem, and become self-efficacious. In summary, utilizing positive performance anxiety is the first step to be motivated to enhance your body esteem quotient (BEQ). Now, let me show you how to tap into that resource.

Break a Leg: Performance Anxiety

I marvel at Pink's performances because she is truly a performer in every sense of the word! If you are wondering if you have seen another artist put more energy into acrobatics high above the audience, you may be thinking of Cirque du Soleil. If you have ever performed in a play, musical, or dance recital, you have probably been told by your cast mates to "break a leg!" Staying motivated for any type of performance is a learned skill and discipline that becomes stronger just by doing it, over and over. No performer would ever miss a rehearsal or show, thus the standard of the industry, "the show must go on." Everyone experiences a certain amount of anxiety (a few butterflies) when they are performing, whether it be at your apprenticeship as a student teacher, board meeting presentation, or a soccer match. Positive anxiety allows you to perform at your peak and does not sabotage your efforts of preparing in advance for the event, unlike negative anxiety that may inhibit your ability to perform well. Athletes refer to the concept of "choking" when the performance does not go as well as one had hoped, and we all have witnessed this at the Olympics; it is heartbreaking to watch when an athlete falls short of their dream after years of blood, sweat, and tears.

Performance anxiety, one of the most common forms of anxiety, can manifest itself in a plethora of ways and plays a significant role in many aspects of our lives such as test taking, speaking engagements, theatrical or musical performances, sports competitions, and career and academic performances. Even asking for a raise can bring on performance anxiety because the result of the answer likely depends on how well you have performed. Psychologists and business mentors can help one overcome these challenges and get back on or stay on track to achieve their ultimate vision!

My clinical impressions are that overachievers are highly motivated due to their self-imposed pressure, perfectionism, and eagerness to please others or achieve personal gain and satisfaction. On the other hand, underachievement can occur due to fear of failure, focusing on past mistakes, and experiencing a loss of risk taking to perform well due to not wanting to feel the sting of disappoint in oneself or by others. Anyone anxious about an upcoming performance or event such as auditions for drill team or a job interview can allow fear to sabotage their effort or experience a sense of past failure and the pain of disappointment. This can absolutely manifest in how one feels about their body. Perhaps you feel compelled to lose weight or become more physically fit due to high levels of anxiety to perform well, and there may be sudden weight loss or gain. How many times have we heard brides say "I have to lose weight before my wedding?" Body image issues can potentially become the manifestation or symptom of an underlying problem such as self-doubt that negatively impacts your body esteem. However, if the positive performance anxiety is channeled productively, it can serve as a motivator to excel.

Moreover, there are many resources at your fingertips to improve your positive performance anxiety and keep you motivated. Negative performance anxiety can adversely affect the outcome of your performance but can be overcome with anxiety reduction techniques, biofeedback, systematic desensitization, and anti-anxiety medications (PQ). Anxiety reduction techniques such as progressive muscle relaxation or guided imagery are available to you online via workbooks, YouTube, or apps. Biofeedback is a technique often used to learn to control your body's functions, such as your heart rate. With biofeedback, you are connected to electric sensors where you receive information about your body. I have seen it work wonders in terms of learning to manage anxiety-provoking situations such as testifying in court or an acting debut. Systematic desensitization is a behavioral technique used to treat fear, anxiety, and phobias. It is similar to exposure therapy; by using this method the person participates in a relaxation exercise and is gradually exposed to an anxiety-producing stimulus, like an object or place. Many of the anti-anxiety medications act as a beta blocker and do not impair cognitive functioning and improve symptoms such as trembling hands or feeling overwhelmed and provide a sense of calmness.

The symptoms of performance anxiety fall under three categories: cognitive, physical, and behavioral. Cognitive anxiety appears to stem from fear of failure that you have not acquired the knowledge and skill, and one overprepares for an event (i.e., compulsively overexercising before a gymnastic competition and injuring oneself). Some of the cognitive symptoms of performance anxiety are as follows: negative self-image or self-evaluation, internal locus of control where failure is always their fault, not comfortable accepting compliments, which seems more common in regards to their body (i.e., "You look great in that outfit" and one responds, "I actually feel fat!"), requirements are unrealistic for themselves, and attempts to avoid anxiety and performance anxiety overwhelms their thought processes.

The physical symptoms may manifest themselves in regard to performance anxiety as follows: face and neck turning red, rapid heart palpitations, stomach or bowel complaints, headaches, hyperventilating, and blackouts. These may be noticeable when one is giving a speech, or taking college entrance exams or state board exams for licensure for becoming a psychologist, physician, beautician, or nurse. The physical symptoms are real and not psychosomatic but can be managed successfully.

The behavioral symptoms of performance anxiety are procrastination, perfectionism, avoiding certain tasks, and daydreaming. Procrastination and avoidant behavior seem to be more common with bulimia nervosa, ADD/ADHD, compulsive overeating, or binge eating disorder because the symptoms of bingeing and/or purging serve as a distractor from the task at hand. The endorphin effect that is received from bingeing and purging reduces stress and anxiety and can become a maladaptive way to cope.

Perhaps you avoid certain tasks because they are not your strongest aptitude, or you are gifted and talented and not intellectually challenged. If it is a mandatory task such as your academic curriculum or a work project, then seek out tutorials or support because the anxiety may be psychological (i.e., fear of failure), or acquire more skills. If you have test anxiety or learning disabilities, which are not a reflection of your intelligence quotient, you may request accommodations such as untimed tests, a different testing format, or a more conducive work environment. A psychoeducational assessment that identifies areas of strength and weakness will improve your academic functioning and career development path. If you are dissatisfied with your career or major, submit your curriculum vita to a headhunter or complete a career assessment (i.e., Strong Interest Inventory and Myers-Briggs Type Indicator, which can be completed online, via some businesses and psychologists) that identifies your job preferences and personality traits that match. Clearly, this will make the assignment more palatable, and you will be more motivated! Implement a positive reinforcement (i.e., Starbuck's gift card) after a laborious task so you reward yourself. Learn to gracefully decline projects that are not enjoyable (i.e., treasurer for a charity when you dislike accounting) and delegate (i.e., hire a bookkeeper or accountant for your taxes). Some of the most successful people have learned the art of delegating and recognizing their strongest aptitudes where they put the majority of their energy.

Motivational Spectrum

Motivational interviewing is used by mental health professionals to assess the level of motivation for their patients. It is a helpful clinical tool that can identify the reasons they may feel stuck and unable to move forward.

I have designed my own assessment for you to identify your level of motivation and the underlying reasons why you may not be motivated. Once you have identified with the aforementioned, the motivational checklist will help you see where you might want to put some of your focus.

Not Motivated/Somewhat Motivated/Motivation Comes and Goes/Highly Motivated

Motivational Checklist:

Move Past Procrastination
Optimize Healthy Interpersonal Relationships
Tackle Cognitive Dissonance
Identify if You Are Intrinsically or Extrinsically Motivated
Validate Yourself and Strive for Self-Efficacy
Allow Deprivation to Motivate You
Take Charge of Your Stress Management
Identify Methods of Enabling or Rescuing
Overcome Roadblocks
No More Learned Helplessness

Facing the Music: **M**ove Past Procrastination

Music therapy is used in our clinics to explore issues like body image and perfectionism. Writing lyrics provides insight on how one thinks, feels, and behaves (PQ). Write your own lyrics or connect with someone else's lyrics as a means to gain insight and express yourself. Learn to "face the music" by identifying the reasons that you may be procrastinating, such as feeling overwhelmed. Sometimes we have difficulty seeing the forest for the trees, so journal your thoughts and feelings and become solution oriented. If you have good intentions to sign up for a water aerobics class but do not act on it, identify the reasons you are procrastinating. Develop a systematic plan of action such as delegating tasks to others and learning to say no to more commitments so that you put yourself first when it comes to your exercise quotient (EQ).

One can learn to move past procrastination and avoidant behavior and become more motivated. I began studying the piano at age thirty-five, and I have literally learned to appreciate the saying "Face the Music." It is more exciting to play measures that I have mastered but more challenging to play the ones that are technically more difficult. As I was learning

Liszt's "Liebersträum" (one of my favorite piano compositions probably because my cat's name is Liszt), my piano teacher recommended I memorize specific measures to increase my speed and to avoid looking at the music and the keyboard. She suggested I purchase glasses that basketball players use to avoid looking down at the ball and to keep their eye on the game. I eventually mastered this by closing my eyes and becoming more confident in playing. Once I face the music, the joy of achieving this accomplishment is well worth the effort and time invested. All in all, the motivational techniques that I have learned from "facing the music" have been instrumental at the keyboard and away from the piano.

Diamonds, Divas, and Drama: Optimize Healthy Interpersonal Relationships

One of my vices is watching reality television, which it can be quite alluring with the fabulous wardrobes, stars dripping in diamonds, and, of course, the drama. It is tempting to get wrapped up in one of the series and binge watch. In the real world it is not as exciting if you have drama in your relationships. Most of us want to live a life with harmonious and loving relationships. Recent studies are equating healthy relationships with body positivity. You have the power to disengage from the emotional turmoil of a dysfunctional relationship and be drama-free. If you are in a conflictual relationship with your family of origin, ex-spouse, partner, or someone in a toxic work environment, it may be more challenging to achieve your goals. Conflicts in relationships, especially with a power and control dynamic, contribute to poor body image and can feel like an emotional rollercoaster ride. Make a commitment to yourself that you will use your mental energy to optimize healthy interpersonal relationships rather than stay in the cycle of drama.

You may be settling for a relationship that is unhealthy due to avoiding the disappointment of another relationship not working out. You have the ability to rewrite the script of your life. Insert what you really want and need into the narrative. Learn to set healthy boundaries, and when others won't respect your boundaries or won't participate in creating healthy options that can lead to a better life, then do not settle for less in your relationships! Your self-worth will improve significantly if you are engaged in relationships that are emotionally enriched (PQ). Your motivation will soar when you have a strong support system, and can extend throughout your lifespan. It is somewhat common to be drawn to conflict or someone who is emotionally unavailable because it is familiar. You may subconsciously gravitate to a partner, work environment, or relationship similar to one's family of origin or life experiences because even though it may be uncomfortable for you, it is also very familiar. Personal growth and development begin when you become cognizant of your choices and change the dynamic to improve not only your relationships, but how you see yourself.

Aretha Franklin was the Queen of Soul and a real-life diva! Liz Smith once made comments about the Bill Blass gown the eighteen-time Grammy Award winner wore in a Fox television special. She wrote "She must know she's too bosomy to wear such clothing, but clearly she just doesn't care what we think, and that attitude is what separates mere stars from true divas." Aretha fired back and said, "How dare you be so presumptuous as to presume you could know my attitudes with respect to anything other than music. Obviously, I have enough of what it takes to wear a bustier, and I haven't had any complaints. When you get to be a noted and respected fashion editor, please let us all know." All I can say is RESPECT: she commanded it, and she got it!

If your partner or family are critical of your body and make hurtful comments, please closely consider why you are tolerating this. It is an impediment to your body esteem and makes every change more difficult. If you are kissing frogs, examine why you are choosing this type of relationship such as a narcissist or a controlling partner. You deserve to be with someone who is supportive, loving, and kind and who encourages you in your endeavors. Why is anyone who professes to care about you or be interested in you being critical of you? Take a personal inventory of each one of your relationships and introduce conflict resolutions skills, boundaries, distance, or terminate the relationship. There are times that you may choose to terminate a relationship with someone who is disrespectful so you can gain self-respect. And, even if there is a process involved in separating yourself, such as asking for a transfer to a different department, the moment you decide to take action, your motivation can kick into gear.

Triangulation is where two people are at war with one another and you are drawn in the middle to resolve the conflict. You are in a no—win situation, and all you can do is set boundaries and remove yourself from this role because the third party becomes the victim. Drawing healthy boundaries is like drawing a line in the sand and requesting that others not cross it. Redirect both parties to one another so they can resolve their differences. Triangulation occurs in a marital system where the child is drawn into parental conflicts, in the work environment, and with friendships, siblings, and other relationships as well. Set yourself free so you can experience the peace of mind and joy that comes from emotionally enriched relationships.

You do not have to stay stuck in any relationship. Many of us truncate our efforts because we are lonely or afraid of being alone. But even that feeling can be recognized and coupled with the thought that being in a loving and supportive relationship is worth pursuing. The healthiest relationship is the one that begins with you where you truly understand your emotional needs, become psychologically introspective, and build positive self-esteem. The investment in yourself will be highly rewarded because there is a tendency for one to seek out partners with the same level of self-esteem. Controlling relationships often grow out of another person asserting their control out of their own perceived inadequacies. Moving toward supportive loving relationships, even though it may be hard to make changes, will bring more motivation with each step forward while being stuck crushes your spirit over time. Relationship satisfaction and happiness occurs when both partners embrace unconditional love, intimacy, trust, and respect. Loving and appreciating your body is a crucial part of loving yourself.

Eat Cake for Breakfast: Tackle Cognitive Dissonance

Have you seen the pajamas that say "Eat Cake for Breakfast?" I am not suggesting that you have cake for breakfast on a daily basis. While some may think it is crazy, I make chocolate chip cheesecake at Thanksgiving and sometimes have it for breakfast the day after with a cup of lemon ginger tea. This is not a "guilty pleasure"; it is simply pleasurable! Having cheesecake for breakfast annually will not wreck my waistline! Cognitive dissonance can be defined as two thoughts that are incongruent with one another resulting in uncertainty. If your methodology is to explore the pros and cons of a dilemma such as eating cheesecake for breakfast and you make a firm decision, then why induce guilt? Just enjoy it. Indecisiveness is a symptom of depression that correlates with body image issues due to perfectionism and worrying about experiencing guilt after eating what is perceived as a forbidden food.

It appears that the majority of us strive to resolve any cognitive dissonance. My piano teacher plays inside of the piano, which is like a harp turned sideways, and although she is a virtuoso concert pianist, I prefer the sound of chords that are not dissonant because it is more pleasing to the ear. Chords and phrases where the minor keys can stand out and some musical styles like rock or jazz thrive on complex minor scales. While music written in major keys sounds bright and cheery, music in minor keys tends to be darker and somewhat melancholy, with chords to match. Minor chords often modulate to major chords in classical music analogous to our pursuit for resolution in our cognitive functioning.

Cognitive dissonance is similar to ambivalence, and it may hinder motivation. Research shows several reasons that we experience cognitive dissonance, including too many options, which can be overwhelming, eagerness to please others, and eliminating rather than choosing. Cognitive dissonance exponentially increases if you have been chastised by others for making a mistake or are not accustomed to being able to "cast your vote." Start with getting in touch with your thoughts and feelings by journaling the pros and cons of the dilemma. Assert yourself in the decision-making process versus harboring resentments because you did not speak up.

Cognitive dissonance can be overcome, and you will be able to be more decisive in regard to the four quotients. Your vote counts, and your input in decision making is meaningful. Do not allow others to micromanage your food intake and be the food police (NQ) or the exercise police (EQ). There is a sense of freedom when you become an independent thinker and have the emotional maturity (which is characteristic of body positivity) to make your own decisions. Learn to trust your judgement, and you will soar in your ability to stay motivated in decision making.

What Floats Your Sailboat?
Identify If You Are Intrinsically or Extrinsically Motivated

Motivation is referred to in the research as either intrinsic motivation, which is internal, and extrinsic motivation, which is external. It is important to identify which type of these motivations most appeal to you. Intrinsic motivation comes from deriving pleasure from within such as reading one of your favorite authors because you enjoy their novels, plots, and character development. Intrinsic motivation may create more autonomy or locus of control, which means that one exercises more control over themselves. If you are intrinsically motivated to derive pleasure from dressing to flatter your figure versus seeking others' approval, it will lead to more body satisfaction (FQ). You will learn to accentuate your assets such as your legs by selecting clothing that you wear with a sense of self-confidence, such as suede leggings or a leather miniskirt. You will become your own stylist (#BYOS) after going through the process of curating your own closet (#CYOC), which will inspire you to stay motivated to take risks. In essence, intrinsic motivation may be more self-fulfilling and last longer due to the sense of pleasure that it brings.

Extrinsic motivation is the opposite of intrinsic in that the individual seeks out a positive reinforcement for the behavior. If you have improved your stress management and self-care (PQ) you reward yourself with a manicure and pedicure at your favorite spa. Unlike intrinsic motivation, extrinsic motivation relies on factors outside of the person (i.e., movie passes) for achieving your objective. A word of caution is that extrinsic motivators may set themselves up to be dependent on others for validation for their self-esteem and body esteem such as seeking out others' appraisal.

Conversely, the idea of the negative reinforcement acts as a consequence and can be motivational to an extrinsically motivated person. If you have your heart set on getting together with friends to watch your favorite team play, setting this up as your reward based on achieving your exercise goals (EQ) may motivate you more. Competition is one aspect of extrinsic motivation because one becomes more competitive to be the winner and not derive as much pleasure from enjoying the actual event. Instead of enjoying running your first 10K race, an extrinsically motivated person may become more motivated to win the race. Whereas, an intrinsic motivator may walk in a local cancer walk to raise awareness and resources against breast cancer because it is a cause that is near and dear to his or her heart. I encourage you to take one of the assessments online to learn if you are intrinsically or extrinsically motivated so you have a better understanding of how to stay motivated.

The Winner Takes It All:
Validate Yourself and Strive for Self-Efficacy

I love the musical and movie of the rendition of Abba's "Mama Mia!" One of my favorite songs is "The Winner Takes It All." My husband and I saw the musical when it first came out in London, and everyone was drinking champagne and dancing in the aisles. There is now a dinner theater in London where the set is similar to *Mama Mia*, and aspiring Broadway actresses serenade you to songs while you dine! My late mother-in-law loved the music so much that she requested that some of the songs be played at her funeral, which was definitely a celebration of her wonderful life! However, there are life lessons to be learned when we do not win, and it is important to learn those lessons as well.

Serena Williams has been deemed the best female athlete of all time. She continues to triumph over obstacles in her career as a professional tennis player, and it has been said that she has fearless motivation to excel. Serena once said, "I really think a champion is defined not by their wins but by how they can recover when they fall." Serena's response to her loss in the 2018 Wimbledon finals was notable. The tennis superstar remained as gracious as ever and acknowledged her opponent, Angelique Kerber, for her outstanding performance. She stated in an interview, "I was really happy to get this far and for all of the moms out there, I was playing for you today, and I tried, but Angelique played really well." What I find most inspirational about Serena is that she underwent a serious surgery after giving birth to her daughter, Olympia just ten months prior to Wimbledon 2018, yet she continued to prepare for the strenuous competition. She has also pushed back on body shaming on social media. Win or lose, my hat goes off to Serena because she is simply the greatest of all time on and off the court.

According to a Stanford University study, perceived self-efficacy is defined as people's beliefs about their capabilities to produce designated levels of performance that exercise influence over events that affect their lives. For example, one believes that they can improve their cholesterol and blood pressure by nutritionally balanced meals and exercise (NQ and EQ). Such core beliefs that you are confident you can overcome an obstacle include cognitive, motivational, affective, and selective processes. In other words, self-efficacy includes how one thinks, feels, behaves, and motivates oneself. Examining what truly motivates you is an often-overlooked factor in gaining momentum toward your goals.

The beauty of self-efficacy is that one does not have to compete with others, but the focus is on being the very best you can possibly be. Marlo Thomas's father, the late Danny Thomas, has a quote I think describes self-efficacy: "I raised you to be a thoroughbred. When thoroughbreds run, they wear blinders to keep their eyes focused straight ahead with no distractions, no other horses. They hear the crowd, but they don't listen. They just run their own race. That's what you have to do. Don't listen to anyone comparing you to me or anyone else. You just run your own race." If you are trying to lose or gain weight for your physical and psychological well-being (PQ), the focus is not on comparing your nutrition (NQ) and exercise (EQ) to others, but on an individualized plan that is right for you.

Imagine feeling content because you no longer turn yourself into a pretzel to please others. What if constant comparison to others and trying to measure up hinders your motivation? What do you suppose it would feel like to only compete with yourself and be the very best version of yourself? If you want to experience a sense of peace and happiness, you may want to consider embracing self-efficacy. When one experiences success and has self-efficacy, they do more than convey positive appraisals. As business managers or leaders, they avoid putting others in situations prematurely where they may fail, and they measure success in terms of self-improvement as opposed to triumph over others. Perhaps this is because they genuinely care about others and no longer feel compelled to seek others' approval but want others to be successful as well.

During high levels of emotional or physiological arousal (anxiety prior to a podcast or Facebook live) they use this to energize themselves versus undermining their goals or performance. Having a strong sense of efficacy is the best way to become motivated due to the personal accomplishment and sense of emotional well-being (PQ). Self-efficacy will propel you to have more self-esteem and self-confidence. You will no longer compare your achievements or body to others in order to achieve body positivity.

People with high self-assurance approach difficult objectives as a challenge to be mastered, not something to be avoided. An efficacious outlook also embraces intrinsic motivation because in the face of failure, they prevail and learn from their experiences and maintain their level of motivation. Their sense of failure is attributed to insufficient effort or lack of knowledge, and they acquire new skills to begin again. In short, failure is not a curse but simply a lesson to be learned that inspires one to learn from past experiences.

JLo to JGlow: **A**llow Deprivation to Motivate You

Do humble beginnings motivate one to excel in life? The research shows that motivation can increase based on your level of deprivation. When Jennifer Lopez was breaking into Hollywood, executives did not embrace her unique beauty. They would encourage her to lose weight and change her look, but they did not know who they were dealing with! She stood firm in her belief, as taught by her mother and grandmother, to love her body— curves and all! I'm certain you have noticed her incredible work ethic as a dancer, singer, actress, producer, and entrepreneur. She now can add to her curriculum vita the Vanguard award and her own makeup line called JGlow inspired by growing up in the Bronx with glowing skin, neutral shades, illuminator, bronzer, and gloss. She seems to be aging backwards, which she attributes to a healthy diet (NQ) and exercise (EQ) and contends that when you take care of yourself you are better able to take care of those you love.

Feeling deprived of motivation is no joking matter! How do we get our mojo back? Suit up and show up because the simple act of putting one foot in front of the other will eventually propel you to become energized. Although it is important to process emotions for our psychological health, limit your pity party (PQ). Research shows that we are more productive to do our work in short time periods, rather than all at once. The Pomodoro Technique is a method that works by doing tasks in twenty-five-minute sessions, with a five minute break between each session. This technique is effective in helping with one's attention span and the ability to commit to a shorter timeframe is not as overwhelming. If your goal is to implement variety to avoid boredom in your meal planning, but you are short on time (NQ), try new recipes, use a new multi-functional cooker to save time, or order groceries or meals online. Get your kids involved by using a family app to delegate tasks, and make it a family affair.

Prepare in advance for your day such as packing your gym bag (EQ), or meet a friend for coffee or lunch to feel connected (PQ) because this sets the stage for a sense of obligation and accountability, which are excellent sources of motivation. Write down not only your goals, but the rationale behind why you have set these goals. If your goal is to avoid obsessionality about your body by limiting social media, write down the rationale to improve body esteem (PQ). Accept how you may feel now and realize that your lack of motivation will change over time. Find a methodology for becoming inspired that works for you, whether it be a support group, positive affirmations, bibliotherapy (i.e., self-help books and apps) journaling, or seeking out professional counseling.

Take Charge of Your Stress Management

> *"The only trouble with being in the rat race is*
> *even if you win, you are still a rat."*
> —Lilly Tomlin

Even though you may be taking active measures to quell your own anxiety and stress, the daily challenges of life still have to be navigated. Perhaps you are experiencing emotional stress, commuter stress, or worry about your future. Most people typically have an increase or decrease in their appetite when they are stressed. Stress could be one of the culprits. It plays a role in weight gain and weight loss. While stress can result in a decrease in appetite at first, long-term "chronic" stress actually boosts your appetite. And because you may be making an attempt to soothe your stress level, you may find that you have more cravings for simple carbohydrates easily found in junk food when you are stressed.

Fight or Flight

I'm sure that you've heard of the survival response known as fight or flight, but you may not know that your body activates this survival mode once you reach a certain stress level. Why? Because your body thinks you've used calories to deal with your stress, even though you haven't, says Pamela Peeke, MD, an assistant professor of medicine at the University of

Maryland. As a result, it thinks you need to replenish those calories, even though you don't. At this stage it is important to reestablish your hunger and fullness cues. The hunger rating scale in the psychology quotient (PQ) chapter is used to recalibrate the connection between brain, body, and hunger. Stress assessments at https://www.stress.org/self-assessment/ are provided from the American Institute of Stress where you can personalize an inventory that meets your needs such as career stress assessments.

Cortisol and Comfort Foods

Levels of "the stress hormone," cortisol, increase when one is experiencing tension and anxiety affecting our decision making and driving that need for comfort food. Mindless eating or disassociating when you are eating can quickly become habit forming. If you are watching television or at your computer screen and not focused on your natural biological cues such as hunger sensation or satiety, you may not be cognizant of the fact that you are overeating or undereating. Consequently, increased levels of the hormone also cause higher insulin levels, your blood sugar drops, and you crave sugar and high fat foods. So instead of a kale salad or a pomegranate, you're more likely to crave desserts like brownies or starchy foods like mac and cheese. That's why they're called "comfort foods." Eating these foods may actually increase serotonin levels in your brain that are depleted when you are stressed, and that is the reason people sometimes become addicted to food.

Jason Perry Block, MD, an assistant professor at Harvard, says eating can be a source of solace and can lower stress. "This happens, in part, because the body releases chemicals in response to food that might have a direct calming effect." Fatty and sugary foods are usually the foods we choose because we love them and often have memories of comfort associated with them. The bottom line? "More stress = more cortisol = higher appetite for junk food = more belly fat," says Shawn M. Talbott, PhD, a nutritional biochemist. Some are genetically predisposed to have more carbohydrate cravings, which is symptomatic of disordered eating and eating disorders. Medications that serve as a carbohydrate inhibitor are effective, but that does not mean you must avoid all carbs because learning to moderate is key. In my clinical experience, once you begin to identify specific stressors such as financial stress and stress warning signals like tension and insomnia, you will began to normalize your food intake. Take a moment to review the stress warning signals in the chart below and identify which ones you may be experiencing whether they be physical, behavioral, emotional, or cognitive symptoms.

Stress Warning Signals			
Physical Symptoms	**Behavioral Symptoms**	**Emotional Symptoms**	**Cognitive Symptoms**
Headaches	Smoking	Crying	Impaired Concentration
Indigestion	Bossiness	Anxiety	Lack of Creativity
Stomach Ache	Negativity	Sadness	Memory Loss
Sweaty Palms	Grinding Teeth	Irritability	Indecisive
Insomnia	Overuse of Alcohol	Feeling Powerlessness	Obsessive Thoughts
Too Much Sleep	Bingeing	Tension	Ruminating Thoughts
Dizziness	Restricting Food	Anger	Worrying
Tight Neck & Shoulders	Substance Abuse	Loneliness	Loss of Sense
Racing Heart	Sex Addiction	Unhappiness	of Humor
Restlessness	Excessive Time on Technology	Fear	Forgetfulness
Fatigue	Mood Swings	Depression	Cognitive Dissonance
Lack of Motivation	Compulsive Behaviors	Boredom	Confused Thoughts

Identify Methods of Enabling or Rescuing

A common misconception is that millennials are lazy and incompetent, but I think it is important to not label a generation. The general consensus seems to be that millennials have been enabled and rescued, which adversely affects their motivation and achievement orientation. *Forbes* reported that millennials can be highly motivated if you make it clear that you care about them. *Harvard Business Review* found that 59 percent of millennials were likely to experience shame when taking a vacation as opposed to 41 percent of employees thirty-five years and older. I do not want anyone to feel shameful, but being competent and taking responsibility is important. As a generation, millennials' strengths include being well-versed in the world of technology that changes so rapidly, having no fear of confronting problems, completing tasks with quality performance, being eager to learn and create new ideas, and desiring sense of purpose and accomplishment above money and fame.

In many respects millennials are like the rest of us in that they want to be passionate about a cause. Communication is crucial when working with millennials, and it is important to speak to them about their interests and goals. A team of individuals who are utilizing their strengths to accomplish a goal are more efficient, effective, and motivated.

Paradoxically, it is important with any generation to assess if one is being enabled or you are acting as the enabler because this can hinder motivation. There is a fine line between counsel and guidance regardless of what role you play, whether it be a parent, CEO, or teacher, and rescuing another person or allowing yourself to be rescued. If you are acting independently and taking responsibility for yourself, you will be more motivated and productive in boosting your body esteem.

If you are a morning person and you prefer to exercise early in the day, make a personal commitment to your health and wellness and do not allow others to deter you by encouraging you to sleep in or stay up late. If you prefer to exercise in the afternoon or evening, stay strong with your exercise commitment and do not allow others to talk you into a happy hour. In summary, make a list of all of the ways that you may be enabling someone or yourself and how this is impacting your body esteem quotient. Methodically list each quotient such as the nutrition quotient (NQ), exercise quotient (EQ), psychological quotient (PQ), and fashion quotient (FQ) and introduce behavioral changes that will allow you to excel without being rescued or enabled.

Set the Stage for Success

Overcome Roadblocks

Setting the stage for success with regard to your body esteem quotient (BEQ) can help one overcome roadblocks. At the onset, regardless of your weight, it is important to confirm medical stability with a comprehensive preventive medical exam. The preventive physical exam and the psychological assessment establish baseline measurements on the status of your overall health. One caveat is that independent of one's size and weight, it is imperative that you are physically and mentally healthy. I have worked with both genders in all shapes and sizes, and the key to wellness, prevention, and body positivity is ruling out any medical or psychological complications (i.e., type 2 diabetes, cardiac complications, bone density, amenorrhea or infertility, depression, anxiety, and eating disorders). We require medical clearance in our clinic as a criterion for the patient to enroll in treatment to protect their health. One can be a size 2 and have serious health problems or a size 12 and be perfectly healthy, or vice versa. It is all about taking responsibility for your mental and physical health regardless of your weight or clothing size. Do not wait another minute! Schedule your preventive medical exam so you can take action and be more motivated to pursue body positivity!

Perhaps your test results will confirm that you are doing a phenomenal job, or there may be room for improvement. Although accountability is important for your mental and physical health, there is a tendency to blame yourself and attribute all of the weight changes to behavioral patterns like diet and exercise. Other precipitating factors may contribute to weight variances and should be considered and ruled out, such as pregnancy, hormonal imbalances, thyroid conditions, mental and medical conditions, and medication side effects. Let's begin by clearing your path by checking off each of the aforementioned factors so that you have a fresh start toward being successful and removing all roadblocks.

What to Expect When You Are Expecting

Domestic engineering is one of the most important careers and roles that one can play. After having a baby, you are going through an adjustment phase and may be experiencing postpartum depression, as many new mothers often do. The question arises of how to get rid of those extra pounds, and if you are experiencing postpartum depression, it may impact your mood and ability to lose weight, so have a conversation with your doctor and seek out the appropriate treatment. You deserve to have a happy and healthy experience with your new precious baby! If you started out at a normal weight and gained the twenty-five to thirty-five pounds your doctor probably recommended, it typically takes a couple of months to get back to your pre-pregnancy weight. However, this may vary due to other variables such as your thyroid, genetic predispositions, and your weight prior to pregnancy. Therefore, it is important to not compare your weight or progress to other new mothers.

If you were carrying extra weight prior to your pregnancy or you put on more weight than your doctor advised, it may take much longer. Some studies show that it can take up to one year to lose the weight, and the baby weight you gained could stay on longer if you do not lose it. "It's very critical that you do get the weight off, because if you don't it has been associated with overweight and obesity fifteen to twenty years later in life," says Debra Krummel, PhD, RD, endowed professor in the University of Cincinnati department of nutrition. Although all new moms are eager to wear their pre-pregnancy clothes, be patient with yourself. Losing the weight healthfully and slowly allows you to maintain a healthy weight range versus rapid weight loss that can easily be regained. If you are unable to lose the weight on your own, you may want to consult with a licensed registered dietitian who can provide support and accountability.

You may be tempted by seeing some celebrities who have gone straight from the delivery room to a size 2 jeans, but it may have not been a healthy approach. "All the magazines ask, 'How did she do it?' The more important question is, 'Why did she do it?'" says Melinda Johnson, MS, RD, registered dietitian and spokeswoman for the American Dietetic Association (ADA). "They do this with very, very strict diets, and a lot of them do it by getting back into activity before their body is really ready for it." Johnson advocates a more gradual approach to weight loss.

"The number one thing new mothers have to have is a certain amount of patience with their body," she says. "It took nine months to get there. It should take at least that long to get back to their fighting weight." Rosie Huntington Whitley reported on ENews that it took her almost a year to get back into feeling comfortable with her body after giving birth to her son, and she said it wasn't a cakewalk. Be gentle and kind to yourself and baby your body just like you are with your newborn!

Hormones and Weight Changes

Research shows that if one anticipates bodily changes that it may be easier to cope with these issues. For example, 90 percent of women experience weight gain between the ages of thirty-five and fifty-five, not coincidentally, during perimenopause and menopause. One method to counteract this weight gain is to increase your aerobic activity (EQ) and consume calories within your metabolic rate (NQ). Avoid chronic dieting, which can make you more vulnerable for a weight gain later. A preventive and proactive plan will equip you with the tools you need for success, but it may require more effort such as extending your workout time. But, after the age of thirty-five, it is critically important to incorporate healthy nutrition and an exercise prescription and balance your hormones. As your age progresses, your hormones may not be regulated properly, but you can systematically measure the imbalance that perimenopause and menopause cause through your blood work. This is necessary for your psychological and physical health. And why shouldn't you enjoy Act II as much or more than Act I!

Properly balanced hormones can help you maintain or prevent a weight gain. Unbalanced hormones make you prone to gain weight, especially with too much cortisol or too little progesterone, testosterone, or estrogen. The average weight gain is gradual, about ten to fifteen pounds starting in perimenopause and averaging to about a pound a year. However, women who experience early menopause as a result of surgical menopause (hysterectomy) tend to gain the weight at an even more accelerated pace. Trust me because I speak from life experiences, as I was diagnosed with endometriosis and had corrective surgery at age twenty, a hysterectomy at age twenty-one, and my ovaries were removed at age twenty-three. I have been on hormone replacement therapy since then and later had two more surgeries to remove endometriosis and scar tissue. I was recently diagnosed with hypothyroidism, so having my hormones and thyroid checked is important. My personal experiences have allowed me to be more empathetic and acquire the knowledge I need to educate myself and others on the significance of hormonal balance as it relates to body esteem.

According to my husband Philip, who has a clinical expertise in the lifespan of the female fat cell, menopausal weight gain tends to be located on your abdomen as opposed to your hips, thighs, or rear. He contends that there is an enzyme that carries the fat to the abdominal area. But have no fear; you can develop a plan, prepare, and outsmart this change in your body. Proper hormone replacement is your friend, can make you feel fantastic and vital as you age, and certainly can tip the scales in your favor. Strive to avoid the hormone fluctuations in perimenopause that directly impact your mood, appetite, fat storage, and metabolism. That is a thumb's up like for you as you age gracefully!

Our nutrition constitutes 70 percent of our physical well-being, exercise and quality of life is approximately 25 percent, and the hormones are 5 percent. However, if your hormones are unbalanced, this will impact your overall health. You would never expect to retire without enough wealth to live comfortably without some sort of plan and attention. Similarly, it is the same with your body. I firmly believe that health is the new wealth for our future! Seek out a treatment plan with a gynecologist who is skilled in hormone regulation and can objectively measure your hormone levels through your bloodwork rather than a doctor who provides a random prescription based on norms that may not be the exact dosage for your body.

The English Rose: No More Learned Helplessness

Change is scary for many of us, and becoming psychologically introspective is helpful during times of transition. Having an optimistic, positive perspective regarding life's challenges, you are more likely to overcome them. You will become more proactive rather than reactive, motivated rather than discouraged, and confident rather than anxious.

There are three beliefs that characterize a pessimistic way of thinking rather than an optimistic one: Permanence—the belief that problems are permanent and will never end. Pervasiveness—the belief that problems are all encompassing and universal. Personalization—The belief that all problems come internally from you. Conversely, an optimist's cognitions are as follows: Problems are temporary and can be resolved. Problems are particular to that event/person/experience, not related to everything. Problems are external and not a reflection of who you are.

Learned helplessness is a condition in which a person suffers from a sense of powerlessness, arising from a traumatic event or persistent failure to succeed. Feeling powerless over life circumstances is characteristic of disordered eating or an eating disorder because those engaged in eating this way feel that food is one thing they can control. However, if one succumbs to failure as their fate, they may overlook opportunities to find solutions to the problem. The research shows that learned helplessness is associated with psychological disorders and can exacerbate depression, anxiety, phobias, loneliness, and shyness, which is a genetic predisposition. Social anxiety is often found with disordered eating or eating disorders, but learning social skills and having success in a social environment like a holiday party will help anyone feel more empowered (PQ).

Studies reveal that explanatory styles play a significant role in determining how people are affected by learned helplessness. If your explanatory style is to have a positive mental attitude, this will decrease the likelihood for learned helplessness and act as a deterrent. An effective strategic plan to combat learned helplessness involves cognitive, emotional, and behavioral techniques. Take a moment and list all of the areas of your life where you feel powerless and then write down three plans (A, B, and C) on how to counteract and cope with these issues and implement change and act on them (PQ).

Kathy Lee Gifford is a talented co-host, comedian, songwriter, singer, author, actress, philanthropist, and entrepreneur who can now add to her resume a wine label and film producer. Her husband, Frank Gifford died a few years ago, and I have been amazed at how she has gracefully worked through this loss. She often refers to this time in her life as a wonderful season, and she is a testament of how one can prevail with an optimistic attitude and hope for the future.

Working through the grief cycle after the death of a loved one can be quite challenging, but achievable. Being motivated to move forward can diminish the emotional suffering of grief and bereavement. It does not mean you have forgotten about that person because you will always have cherished memories. Life is filled with changes and profound losses, and it is sad to say our goodbyes whether they be to a loved one or closing a chapter in our life. It is important to grieve our losses and put closure on them so we can move forward and embrace new experiences. Once we go through the bereavement cycle, we make room for new adventures and open ourselves up for new discoveries that perhaps we never dreamed would happen.

My mother-in-law was a lovely English lady who adored roses. She called one day and was very tearful and said, "He died suddenly, and we buried him in the back garden." At the time I was relatively new in the family and wondered if this was a British custom to bury loved ones in their gardens. I assumed it was my father-in-law and offered to call my husband to give him the news. She went on to say that Peter, my father-in-law, bought the new CD *Time to Say Goodbye* by Andrea Bocelli and Sarah Brightman, and they both had a cry about Barley, their beloved English lab that was buried in the back garden. Needless to say, I was relieved that it was not my father-in-law but saddened by the fact that Barley had passed away.

As cliché as it sounds, time heals most wounds, and one day your sadness will be replaced with joy. It takes approximately two years to overcome the grief and bereavement cycle, which is shock and denial, depression, anger, bargaining, and acceptance. Shortly after I started working on this book, my mother passed away. I had the opportunity to tell her that I planned to dedicate this book to her since she was my biggest fan. Her response was, "Well, if you are going to dedicate it to me, it damn well better be a *New York Times* number-one bestseller!" My mother was a hoot and had a heart of gold! This memory is bittersweet, but her words of encouragement and the fact that she taught me to overcome my fears, believe in myself, and pursue my dreams inspires me to be the best author I can possibly be! Mother, this book is for you and how you encouraged me to share my knowledge to help others learn to love their bodies! I will always love you, which was also your favorite song!

Chapter 2
Psychology: Peace of Mind

"What lies behind you and what lies before you
pales in comparison to what lies inside of you."
—Ralph Waldo Emerson

When I grew up in a small town in Texas, one of the traditions that I experienced as a child at my school was an annual Halloween festival. I remember that one of my favorite activities was the cakewalk where you could win a homemade cake if you landed on the right spot in a circle once the music stopped. Hence, the saying "piece of cake," which means a surprisingly easy task. The British have an expression, referring to things as "easy peasy." However, life is not always a cakewalk! In fact, the healthiest individuals are subjected to experiences that may impact their emotional well-being and body esteem. The techniques in this chapter will act as a navigation system and guide you on how to maintain body positivity through life's most challenging obstacle course.

As you have read, we are going to take on the four quotients of body esteem, and we will start with psychological health. We all deserve "peace of mind" and to live life to the fullest. As a psychotherapist and clinical director, I have observed that human beings are incredibly resilient. Moreover, we have the capacity to foster emotional strength and endurance to overcome life's challenges! But we can also be emotionally vulnerable about the things we most care about. Our body image is often a struggle, as we truly want to be confident and believe we are worthy, yet we often find people who barely know us or don't know us at all to judge us on our presentation, including but certainly not limited to, our physical appearance. This may precipitate feelings of inadequacy if we allow others' criticism about our body to define how we see ourselves. Learning to view your body through your own lens is the first step to enhancing body esteem. Historically, many of us have looked to body type trends throughout the decades to emulate, but I am suggesting a more current yet long-term approach to body esteem that embraces our individuality.

Figure Fads Over the Decades

Let's take a trip down memory lane and look at what has been in vogue with regard to figure types and why body esteem is so relevant to mental health. One article revealed that the "ideal woman" has had her silhouette put through a series of fun house mirrors. It changes almost as much as fashion in that the physical qualities that we embrace today may be gone tomorrow. And bodies just don't change that much or that often, yet we try to mold our own body into whatever is most in fashion at the time, often going against our physique and body type. In the 1940s the military shoulders and pointed bras referred to as "bullet" bras were fashionable and a reflection of World War II. Fast forward to the '50s, which was the decade of the hourglass figure. *Playboy* magazine and Barbie emerged during this decade, and a small waist and perfectly perky large breasts were emphasized. The '60s reflected the motto that "thin is in," and an androgynous figure was to be celebrated with no more girdles. Weight Watchers was founded in 1963 because more women wanted to diet to achieve this body type. The '70s era of discotheques, bellbottoms, and platform shoes maintained that the ideal body was still lean, but curvy hips were popular again. The '80s introduced the fitness era, which was a step in the right direction, but many women felt enormous pressure to not only be thin but fit as well. This is when ageism began in that women of all ages were being held to the same standard of fitness representing youth. The '90s introduced the waif look and a disturbing trend known as "heroin chic." As we approached the millennium, a lean but curvaceous body was the ideal look, and Victoria Secret's lingerie dominated the runway. In the 2000s booties became all the rage, and eventually you could actually purchase a "butt bra" for extra padding. One of the newest trends for women in swimsuits is to capture a pose called "Barbie feet" where you point and stand on your tippy toes in hopes of giving the illusion that you are taller and more slender.

Let me recap the figure fads over the decades: breasts that can be pointed like Madonna's Blonde Ambition tour to androgynous breasts, a voluptuous figure that can be modified to a "thin is in" body type, a waif look that has to suddenly become more physically fit, and buttocks that can go from flat to nicely rounded. The relevance of this historical account is to be cognizant of the fact that the societal norms for the "perfect figure" are ever-changing, unrealistic, and unobtainable.

Research shows that a core component of individual body dissatisfaction is appearance-based social comparisons. One becomes dissatisfied with their body when you compare your own body to others. Women are particularly biased to spontaneously direct their attention to the bodies of thin women. It can be daunting to try to become whatever is currently popular. An essential fundamental of body esteem is to not get sucked into allowing any "ideal body" image to affect how you see yourself. A more modern and sustainable approach is to take care of ourselves and build a strong, resilient, and attractive body on our own terms, which includes taking responsibility for your physical and mental health. Your body is uniquely yours, and as such, an incredible part of expressing your autonomy is through your unique physicality. By embracing your physical body, you can begin to integrate your psychological well-being on the way to being whole.

Icing on the Cake

My mother was an incredible baker who made homemade cakes like carrot cake, strawberry cake, and German chocolate cake from scratch. As kids, we loved to lick the delicious unused icing from the beaters and bowl. The psychological quotient is foundational to building better body esteem. It is the cake before the icing. Without a sound psychological structure, other efforts will fall flat or still not deliver any peace, regardless of the effort or outcome. It is imperative that your mind and spirit engage positively with your body in order to have body esteem. The other quotients such as exercise, fashion, and nutrition will be explored later. With that said, it is important to establish healthy psychological functioning in order to savor the icing on the cake. Emotional stability and regulation are the foundation from which you can build upon with the other quotients. Once you have improved your psychological quotient, the others will add delight and a deliciousness to who you are and the uniqueness of what only you can offer, the "icing on the cake."

Emotional Eating Assessment

Please answer the following questions **True** or **False** and score your test afterwards.

1. I eat when I am not hungry.
2. I do not register hunger sensation or satiety.
3. I can differentiate between physical hunger and emotional hunger.
4. I eat when I experience emotions like loneliness, boredom, stress, depression, or anxiety.
5. I accept the fact that I do not have to have the perfect body.
6. I prefer to eat alone because I feel embarrassed or ashamed.
7. My family and friends make negative comments about my food intake and try to control how much or what I am eating.
8. I typically experience guilt or shame after eating what I perceive as a forbidden food such as desserts.
9. I am emotionally mature, and my chronological age matches my level of maturation.
10. I think about my weight most of the time and worry that I will gain weight.
11. For the most part I like my body, and I exercise and eat healthfully.
12. I sometimes skip meals, fast, restrict, binge, purge, take laxatives or diuretics, or overexercise.
13. I feel physically fit, and I am comfortable with the way that I look in my clothes.

14. When a problem arises, it derails my eating habits, and I tend to overeat or undereat.
15. I am very concerned about what others think of my body, and I try to please them.
16. I stress over the responsibilities of adulthood and have difficulty managing issues like finances, balancing career and personal life, and parenthood.
17. I embrace intimacy and can handle rejection and have rewarding relationships.
18. I am not conflict avoidant and feel comfortable asserting myself when I am upset.
19. I am hopeful about my future and improving my quality of life.
20. I have a strong support system, and I feel comfortable seeking help in times of need.

You can find the scoring key at www.bodyesteem.com

The Best Gift You Can Give Yourself: Self-Esteem

Clearly, we may never look like the supermodel Gisele Bundchen or Michangelo's David. Body image is a complex phenomenon, and there are many factors that lead to body dissatisfaction: weight gain, paradoxical messages from the media and constant access to social media, cultural pressures, perfectionism, drive for thinness, low self-esteem, being in a relationship where a loved one is disapproving, abandonment through loss or divorce, emotional immaturity, delayed psychosexual development (e.g., never been kissed), mood swings, loss of control, trauma, physiological changes such as hormonal imbalances or pregnancy, chronic illness, disfigurement (e.g., breast mastectomy), sexual abuse, sexual misconduct, and sexual harassment. Regardless of the reasons you may struggle with body image, I am confident in your ability to optimize your psychological health.

Self-esteem is critically important to overcoming body image issues. Eleanor Roosevelt once said, "Nobody can make you feel inferior without your consent." If we respond to others with the statement "You make me feel . . ." we are giving up our emotional power. We are responsible for our own emotional state, and emotions are not contagious. If someone makes a negative comment about your body, you do not have to allow this to affect how you feel about yourself. Self-esteem is defined as a confidence and satisfaction in oneself: self-respect. Self-esteem is the greatest gift that you can give yourself because you control it, and it cannot be bought or stolen if you value and safeguard it. I saw an adorable hand towel that read, "Whatever . . . I'm Still Fabulous." I'm not advocating being dismissive about constructive feedback, but I do wholeheartedly believe that you alone are in charge of your self-esteem. It is okay if you feel like your self-esteem isn't where you want it to be. Part of the purpose of this chapter is to connect with how you currently feel about your body, how much of your power you are giving to others, including the images you see through both traditional and social media, and how you process your thoughts about your body. I believe that you do not need to broadcast to the world that you have good self-esteem, but simply exude a level of self-confidence. You can have positive self-esteem and still be thoughtful and kind without being self-absorbed or narcissistic. In fact, greater self-esteem can help you be more generous without the constant worry about what others will think.

Cry Baby Cry

Have you ever felt like you wanted to cry but held back your tears? Emotional stability permeates all parts of our lives, and you can manage your emotions effectively. There are gender differences when it comes to expressing our emotions. Ad Vingerhoets is a Dutch clinical psychologist and author of the book *Why Only Humans Weep: Unravelling the Mysteries of Tears.* His work suggests the stereotype about women crying more than men is actually true: women cry thirty to sixty-four times a year, whereas men cry just six to seventeen times per year. Since his research is self-reported, he contends that men could be underreporting. According to Vingerhoets, we can intuit that men cry less often than women due to social conditioning and stereotypical manhood image. Men may also be biologically designed to shed fewer tears because male hormones like testosterone inhibit crying. Emotional tears contain serum prolactin levels, a hormone produced by the pituitary gland that is associated with emotions, and adult women have 60 percent higher levels than adult males.

Interestingly enough the serum prolactin levels are almost equal for both genders during puberty when hormones are flying high.

Somewhere along the way we began to feel embarrassment about crying and began to suppress our tears because we believe that perhaps it is a sign of weakness. Crying can be therapeutic as a means to express our sorrow and nurture ourselves. Learning to not suppress your emotions is crucial for overcoming emotional eating and body esteem. Studies show that crying has some physical and psychological benefits: it has a self-soothing effect, calms oneself, reduces distress, and regulates emotions. Crying activates the parasympathetic nervous system (PNS), which helps people relax.

I propose that we not only stop body shaming but no longer judge someone if they become emotional or tearful. "Cry, baby, cry" because there is no shame in expressing emotions, and in fact it leads to a healthy psychological quotient (PQ). Most of all, begin to notice when you label crying as negative and say things like, "I don't know why I'm crying" or "This shouldn't have upset me so much." Let your tears provide the needed release and soothe yourself. On the other hand, if you find yourself sobbing uncontrollably for prolonged periods of time, you may want to seek out professional counseling because this could potentially be symptomatic of depression or another psychological issue.

Bowl of Spaghetti:
Emotions, Cognitions, and Behaviors

Emotional regulation is key when it comes to managing our emotions, cognitions, and behavior. All three go hand in hand and are interwoven like a bowl of spaghetti. I bought a pink pasta holder at a kitchen store in Sandwich, England, years ago. When you grab a handful of pasta to add to the pot, it is untangled and straight, and it becomes intertwined when you drain it or add it to the sauce. Emotional eating is a form of disordered eating and is defined as "an increase in food intake in response to negative emotions." It is an unhealthy strategy used to cope with unpleasant feelings. Emotional eaters are at high risk for binge eating disorder, disordered eating, and formal eating disorders. It is paramount to identify emotional dysregulation to avoid eating difficulties.

Emotional regulation is where one is in touch with their emotions and becomes cognizant of their feelings at the time they are experiencing them. Our emotions will be heard one way or another, and if not expressed in a productive way, can manifest through our eating habits or other maladaptive behaviors such as spending excessive time on technology or overspending. The wonderful books written about emotional intelligence explain how someone can have a high intelligence quotient (IQ), but be lacking in their emotional intelligence (EQ). One may perform well in their career and academic situations but have not learned the skill of being psychologically introspective. If someone has poor impulse control when it comes to shopping, eating, and drinking, this may adversely affect their body image. There may be a tendency to overspend to accommodate weight variances as a result of overeating or drinking excessively. All three exacerbate one another, but you can overcome this. As you learn to improve your psychological quotient (PQ) by understanding your emotions, cognitions, and behaviors, you will increase body esteem.

Cognition is a term referring to the mental processes involved in gaining knowledge and comprehension. These processes include thinking, knowing, remembering, judging, and problem-solving. These are higher level functions of the brain that encompass language, imagination, perception, and planning. Most people who struggle with emotional eating are highly functioning individuals and respond well to cognitive behavior therapy. In fact, patients who have an eating disorder have a higher IQ than the normal population. One caveat is if one is experiencing a nutritional deficit such as lack of protein to the brain, it impacts their cognitive functioning and ability to think rationally. Once one normalizes their eating style, their thought processes are restored.

The definition of behavior in the field of psychology consists of an organism's external reaction to its environment. In regard to behavioral patterns with emotional eating, it is more common for someone to seek out treatment when their behaviors are no longer manageable. Behavior modification can be very beneficial such as implementing strategies like attending cooking classes taught by a registered dietitian and learning to overcome your fear of forbidden foods such as carbohydrates.

What's Eating You?

Emojis have become a means of communication on how one expresses their emotions through social media. My personal favorites are the musical notes, staff, and symbols for a piano keyboard since I love playing the piano. Others have favorites that express affection, opinion, or even sadness. There is actually an emoji day, and apparently the most used ones are the smiling faces or the sad faces with tears. Emojis have been embraced as a quick and easy way to communicate emotion. Often, our emotions show up in how we relate to our physical body.

The therapeutic technique of learning to identify emotions and how they correlate with your eating habits is a learned behavior. Interoceptive awareness is a psychological term that is used to describe how one has difficulty recognizing and accurately responding to emotional states such as boredom. Furthermore, it indicates some confusion in the identification of certain visceral sensations related to hunger and satiety. Learn to identify your emotions as part of observing your eating patterns by using the hunger rating scale below, and you will normalize your eating style.

Hunger Rating Scale

Ravenous/Hunger Sensation/Still Hungry/Comfortably Full/Exceed Satiety

Emotions Prior to Eating

Emotions During the Eating Process

Emotions after Food Intake

Perhaps something is bothering you and you cannot quite put your finger on what it is. Research shows that one typically copes with emotions as follows: avoidant coping (i.e., procrastinating or not facing the issue due to fear or anxiety), emotion-focused coping (i.e., using food as a substance to sedate emotions like loneliness), and problem-focused coping (creating a rational plan). Emotional eating typically falls into avoidant coping or emotion-focused coping or both, which are counterproductive. With that said, learning to implement a strategic plan in advance for potential eating complications is effective. If you know you are attending a five-course wedding reception, plan in advance how you will manage the courses. Peruse the menu and consume the courses that you enjoy the most first so you will please your palette. Once you become more aware of how your emotions are affecting what you eat, you can register hunger sensation and satiety.

Psychological Quotient (PQ): The best approach for managing your emotional eating is problem-focused coping, which is a rational plan where you implement a strategy in advance for potential challenges that may arise.

What's Normal?

When it comes to nutrition as it relates to our psychological functioning, the question always arises as to what is normal or abnormal. There really isn't any one thing that is "normal," but becoming normalized is operating within a spectrum with a midpoint and two end points. Many factors and behaviors make up this spectrum. Our eating patterns become habitual behaviors over time due to our lifestyle and personal circumstances and eventually define the type of eater you have become. Our cognition and emotions do impact our behaviors, and all of them are closely related. If you are obsessing about your food, especially carbohydrates, you may develop feelings such as fear of gaining weight, which ultimately affects your behavior (restricting at one end of the spectrum and overeating at the other end). Maladaptive behaviors drift to the ends of the spectrum and can become your eating style, which affect your nutritional intake.

Normalizing Your Eating: What is considered "normal" in terms of quantities and types of food consumed varies considerably from person to person. "Normal eating" refers to the attitude a person holds in their relationship with food, rather than the type or amount of food they eat. In short, normal eating is flexible and does not allow your emotions to dictate your food intake. It varies in response to your schedule, your hunger sensation, and your proximity to food. In general, you allow food to nourish your body without feeling remorseful or guilty, and you partake of all of the food groups.

Normalized eating is when you:

- Eat more on some days, less on others
- Eat some foods just because they taste good
- Have a positive attitude toward food
- Do not label foods with judgement words such as "good," "bad," or "clean"
- Overeat occasionally
- Undereat occasionally
- Anticipate and look forward to eating versus approaching it with a sense of dread
- Crave certain foods at times
- Treat food and eating as one small part of a balanced life
- Consume all of the food groups
- Eat in accordance with your resting metabolic rate
- Do not experience guilt or remorse after eating
- Consume balanced nutrition and stay in a healthy weight range
- Don't compare your food intake, exercise, weight, or size with others
- Establish the amount of calories your body needs
- Honor your hunger sensation and satiety
- Use your interoceptive awareness: mindful and intuitive eating
- Don't let your emotions rule your food intake
- Differentiate between dehydration and hunger

Finding Your Voice

Kelly Clarkson has captured fans' hearts ever since she won the first season of *American Idol* in 2002 with her virtuoso voice! She now is a judge on *The Voice*, and her delightful personality bubbles over like a bottle of champagne! Despite her abundant talent and cheery disposition, she has been relentlessly scrutinized for her appearance for years. She has certainly been a role model on how one learns to find their voice and express themselves, and she has done so both directly and through her music, as she did when she sang "Whole Lotta Woman" at the Billboard Music Awards. Her candid conversations and lyrics from her songs resonate with anyone who has struggled with body image.

You cannot control what others think of your body or even say about your body, and this can have a significant impact on your emotions. In fact, most people have hypersensitivity about their body being criticized, and it seems it is more hurtful than other types of criticism. Your body is so personal that any criticism cuts deep when we seek approval and validation from others. I propose that we stop engaging in any negative talk about anyone's body. Let's focus instead on more self-respect and mutual respect. The objective is to take back your emotional control and not buy into how others see you. Self-possession and self-preservation are preventive techniques that protect one from unsolicited critical remarks. If you assert yourself when someone is critical of your body and set boundaries, it actively protects you. I have seen many family members who are deeply hurt by friends and family "just being honest," which is code for "just judging you." Similarly, it is equally important to not solicit other's feedback regarding your body (i.e., Do I look like I have gained weight?). If you believe and feel good about their positive feedback, then it follows that you would believe and feel badly about their negative feedback. Throughout this book, I will give you the tools to self-monitor and come to your own conclusions.

Psychological Quotient (PQ): Learn to validate your own self-esteem and body image and not look to others for their endorsement or approval.

Are You Hangry?

Many of us are taught: "Good girls don't get mad, and they certainly don't get jealous!" In fact, the two emotions that women avoid the most are anger and jealousy. According to Merriam-Webster's dictionary *hangry* is defined as: bad-tempered or irritable as a result of hunger. Most girls and women feel guilty if they experience anger and have difficulty recognizing this emotion. If you do not express your anger appropriately, it can be internalized and turn into depression. I refer to this as "swallowing your emotions," which can be manifested through behaviors such as being aggressive, passive-aggressive, or passive. You may have seen this when someone becomes passive-aggressive and gives others the silent treatment or aggressive by being hostile and sabotaging a relationship. In either case, you don't want to be in the path of these maladaptive behaviors. It is important to pick your battles when it comes to conflict resolution. Find your voice by becoming more assertive: lower voice inflection, use "I" statements, and avoid the blaming and shaming game. People who are assertive typically get their needs met, do not suppress emotions, and are more respected by others.

Throughout my career, I have worked with patients who participate in competitive dance such as ballet, ballroom, drill team, and ice dancing. Often times they were considering dropping out of dance due to the tendency to compare their bodies to others. I challenged them to use this opportunity as a dress rehearsal for life lessons since there is a likelihood this will reoccur in the future. The objective was to not allow their emotions to rule their passion for their perspective dances. A study published in the *European Journal of Social Psychology* showed that women who tended to compare themselves to others were most affected by jealousy. Some females experience jealousy that tends to stem from comparison, competition, and the fear of losing a mate or potential partner. Research shows that women tend to be more jealous than men in a range of situations and seem to suffer more from emotional jealousy than from sexual jealousy.

Studies reveal that women are most likely to feel jealous of other women based on physical attractiveness. If you experience anger or jealousy, acknowledge it and do not allow others or yourself to induce guilt; instead process your emotions. Perhaps you are jealous because of insecurities or a fear of not getting things you desire such as wanting to be a bride in lieu of being a bridesmaid. In this example, you may have to become introspective to determine if you have been dating men who are noncommittal or emotionally unavailable. If that is the case and you want to be a wife and create a happy home, you may need to implement change in your dating style, which will ultimately lead you to becoming a beautiful bride! By acknowledging the root of your jealousy, you bring to light your emotions and can create a plan of action versus acting out your feelings, minimizing, or internalizing.

Social Media and Body Image

Social media is known to have a significant impact on our emotions and body image. In my clinical and personal experience it seems that we are more critical of ourselves than others when we are looking at pictures of ourselves. We may have wishful thinking as we compare our images and bodies to other's photos on Facebook or Instagram, but the first thing we notice about our own pictures are our flaws. Perhaps we take it one step further and validate our self-esteem and body image based on how many "likes" and comments we receive. As social media evolves, the popularity of photo-based platforms like Instagram and Facebook, which feature front-faced camera selfies, video clips, and enhancements, continues to soar.

It is wonderful that we can capture a memory in a moment's notice and record pictures of friends and family for special events. Historically, these pictures were not shared as widely or as frequently with others except with close friends and family in a more intimate setting. Today technology allows us to see ourselves and others instantaneously without delaying gratification. Although this is an amazing advancement, it may create more obsessionality about your appearance and comparative analysis with others.

Dr. Ramani Durasula, a professor of psychology at California State University, defines a *selfie addiction* as "when a person is almost obsessively taking selfies, multiple times a day, and posting on social media." This has been dubbed "selfitis," and it is said to negatively affect body image as social media can attract individuals who are emotionally vulnerable with low self-esteem who are seeking validation.

Does this mean you can never post another picture on social media? Absolutely not! Set the standard for yourself that you will limit the amount of time you spend comparing yourself to celebrities or others or critiquing yourself on social media. Perhaps consider blocking or limiting exposure to certain aspects of social media (i.e., a fashion show with super-thin models) that create obsessionality.

Psychological Quotient (PQ): Limit the amount of time that you spend on social media, and vet posts that create more obsessionality to avoid scrutinizing yourself and comparative analysis in order to build better body esteem.

Emotions Take the Cake

A former patient said her case must "take the cake" because her comorbid diagnoses were depression and bulimia nervosa. As I stated earlier, there is a strong correlation between food and feelings, and a study completed at the University of Maryland revealed that 75 percent of overeating is caused by emotions. There is a tendency for highly functioning individuals to minimize, deny, or intellectualize their emotions. David Burns, MD, the author of the book *Feeling Good*, contends that depression is like the common cold of psychiatric disturbances. One out of four women will experience depression in their lifetime and are twice as likely to become depressed as men, but it is treatable. If you have a cold or flu, you would go to the doctor to seek out treatment. You would rest, drink more fluids, and likely limit your exposure to others for a brief bit. Your psychological health is as important as your physical health, and you can declare a mental health day where you watch movies and hang out in your PJs so you recharge your batteries. It is actually quite common in my profession as a private practitioner to avoid burnout. Some employers even offer paid mental health days along with other benefits. You can overcome emotional eating by becoming psychologically sophisticated and introspective. This will help you to connect the dots between emotions, cognitions, and behaviors.

If you are a fan of Chrissy Metz on the series *This Is Us*, you know her character, Kate struggles with body image, and it is sometimes painful to watch her struggles. Chrissy recently wrote a book called *This Is Me* in which her fun-loving personality is evident. There are many underlying psychological factors that correlate with emotional eating and poor body image. Individuals preoccupied with their weight report their eating pattern or weight interferes with their relationships, career, ability to take risks, and self-esteem. This dynamic has been characteristic of Chrissy Metz's character Kate in her romantic relationship with another character, Toby. Their portrayal of this challenge exemplifies how some overcompensate by going above and beyond the call of duty craving acceptance and a sense of belonging. Relationships are kept at arm's length due to fear of intimacy and fear of rejection. The fact that studies reveal that people who are overweight or obese are often discriminated against in the workplace only compounds the problem. On a more positive note, when a healthy relationship with food is established along with establishing body esteem, relationships flourish.

Studies show that binge-eating disorder indicates that certain individual's binge eating may be triggered by dysphoric moods, stress, depression, and anxiety. The potential to become addicted to the bingeing often acts as a mood elevation or stabilization. There is a tendency for one who is bingeing to avoid social or professional events and to harbor anger or resentment. It appears that the anger and resentment are more self-induced due to perceived failures such as not being able to lose weight or body shaming. Binge-eaters report higher rates of self-loathing, depression, anxiety, somatic concern, interpersonal sensitivity, and disgust about their body size. The bingeing pattern may become a vicious cycle where the binge episode is used to cope with emotions, and while it provides an endorphin effect, afterwards one experiences remorse, guilt, or shame. The dependency on simple carbohydrates elevates the serotonin levels in the brain and suppresses these unpleasant emotions.

Whether it be the moody blues or different spectrums to the degree of emotional eating you're engaging in, you are not alone. Instead of being self-punitive regarding your behavioral patterns, learn to process your emotions and not self-sabotage yourself with emotional eating. People who experience these issues are intelligent, caring, successful, and competent people who can overcome emotional eating. They are fully capable of successful relationships, starting their own businesses, and taking risks. The emotional concepts below and the psychological quotients will provide a better understanding of how our emotions impact our body esteem.

Emotional Unavailability: One surrounds themselves around others who are emotionally unavailable and experiences loneliness, fear of intimacy, and fear of rejection, which leads to unhealthy eating habits. Example: "I tend to date someone who cannot make a commitment or is narcissistic."

Psychological Quotient (PQ): Examine the reasons that you may seek out an emotionally unavailable partner and only settle for more not less in your relationships.

Emotional Hangover: One experiences the aftermath of emotions from an anxiety-provoking or emotionally charged event. Example: "I ate a pint of mint chocolate chip ice cream every night after the breakup with my boyfriend."

Psychological Quotient (PQ): Learn to identify and process your emotions as they occur and apply the hunger rating scale as a tool for mastery.

Flirtatious Food: One is very fearful of consuming too many calories and flirts with food by picking at it, and fear of forbidden foods or weight gain rule your food intake. Example: "Every time I go out to dinner I study the menu in advance online because I am afraid that I will gain weight."

Psychological Quotient (PQ): Practice meal therapy, which is a technique where you systematically calculate the caloric intake of your meal and later transition to trusting yourself to become a more mindful and intuitive eater. Make a list of your fear foods and identify why you are afraid of them after reading the nutrition quotient (NQ) chapter.

Excessive Emotional Eating: One has difficulty identifying emotions and consumes food based on negative emotions because the food itself or the amount of food consumed tends to numb one's feelings. Example: "I often eat pizza when I am not hungry and later experience remorse and guilt."

Psychological Quotient (PQ): Complete the assessment on emotional eating and hunger rating scale as a means to learn to identify your emotions as it relates to your food intake.

Emotional Empowerment: One begins to identify emotions as they occur and feels empowered to process these emotions. Example: "I can assert myself when someone does not respect my boundaries, and if conflict arises, I am confident I can resolve this with others."

Psychological Quotient (PQ): Learning conflict resolution skills and becoming assertive is a means of taking care of yourself and maintaining healthy relationships.

Rational Emotive Eating: Eating when you experience physical hunger and not emotional hunger. Staying in the moment when you are eating and incorporating all of the food groups into your caloric intake. Example: "I consume all of the food groups on the food pyramid and eat when I experience hunger and stop when I am full."

Psychological Quotient (PQ): Keep distinguishing between physiological hunger and psychological hunger and incorporate all of the food groups.

Have Your Cake and Eat It Too!

Can we actually have our cake and eat it too? We may not be able to have it all, but it is certainly possible to balance your food intake and satisfy your cravings. Why do most people enjoy eating? Specific food cravings are unique to our gender and may result in a positive effect on one's mood. Serotonin is a chemical released in the brain after eating carbohydrates that transmits mood stability. Similarly, endorphins are chemicals released after eating fat and chocolate that result in a food-induced euphoric state. Women are more likely to crave chocolate, bread, and ice cream, whereas men are more likely to crave meat, pizza, and potatoes.

Research shows that some of us are genetically predisposed to have more significant cravings for carbohydrates and actually may have a reduction in serotonin. Those "feel good" hormones that we refer to as an endorphin effect can actually be released in the brain when one is experiencing a pleasurable meal like your favorite homemade lasagna or pad thai. One can learn to moderate food cravings and stabilize mood by balancing food intake and avoiding emotional deprivation. Thus, food deprivation (i.e., restrictive diets where you omit your favorite foods or food groups) may create more problems in terms of overeating and bingeing episodes.

If we deprive ourselves of the foods that we love like pasta this may lead to emotional eating and food deprivation. Why do most of us love chocolate? Aside from the velvety silky texture, delectable taste, and the serotonin upsurge, many women crave chocolate prior or during their menstrual cycle due to the reduction in magnesium. The balancing act is to learn to moderate your food intake or your cravings without feeling deprived. Approximately 80 percent of us feel deprived, which leads to bingeing or compulsive overeating. Therefore, pleasing your palette and satisfying those cravings without sabotaging your healthy weight range is obtainable. Emotional eating can lead to overeating, but that does not mean that you have to avoid carbohydrates or the foods that you enjoy. In fact, it is just the opposite because if you satisfy your cravings and eat within your metabolic rate range, it prevents you from overeating. Unless there is a medical diagnosis like diabetes or cardiac complications or a food allergy, one can eat foods you crave in moderation. The good news is that one can learn to control their cravings and occasionally enjoy their Godiva chocolates too!

Psychological Quotient (PQ): Incorporate your favorite foods that you crave in moderation within your caloric intake to avoid feeling deprived and overeating as a result.

Cognitions: Mental Fitness

Cognitive fitness is equally as important as physical fitness and essential to maintain healthy cognitive functioning. According to Harvard Medical School, cognitive fitness embraces memory recall, thinking, learning, recognition, communication, and sound decision making. Cognitive fitness can provide an autonomous and rewarding life. One can learn to build "cognitive reserve" and provide security for a long-term mental fitness. According to this study doctors have identified six steps: optimal nutrition, exercise, stress reduction, social interaction, sleep, and stimulating activities. Make a commitment to yourself to prolong years of mental vitality.

Cognitive behavior therapy is commonly used with patients who have disordered eating or a formal eating disorder. The most common thought processes that lead to cognitive distortions are the ones I developed through my clinical practice. Cognitive distortions may cause irrational thought processes. One can learn to restructure their cognitions by reframing the way that you process information. Once you change your cognitions, your emotions and behavior will follow suit, and you are well on your way to improving your body image.

Dichotomous Thinking: Issues are often seen as black or white with no room for moderation and one thinks in terms of extremes when problem solving. Example: "If I start eating those cookies I will not stop."

Psychological Quotient (PQ): Extreme thought patterns often lead to indecisiveness when it comes to decision making. Learning to moderate your food intake and not overindulge alleviates dichotomous thinking.

Obsessive Compulsive Thinking: Ruminating thoughts dominate your cognitions, which leads to compulsive behaviors. Example: "I worry about how many calories I consume, so I count every morsel I put in my mouth."

Psychological Quotient (PQ): Obsessive compulsive cognitions may zap your mental energy, and there may be minimal room for thought-provoking subjects or a creative temperament.

Crystal Ball: There is a tendency to predict the future without sufficient evidence to draw conclusions. "I know I will never get married because I am too fat."

Psychological Quotient (PQ): If one is spending time projecting into the future, one may not be living in the present. Mindreading or drawing conclusions without valid information can lead to assumptions and the wrong conclusion.

Compare and Contrast Cognitions: A comparative analysis is made with others where you evaluate how much they eat, exercise, and compare your body to others. Example: "I am going to eat and exercise as much as the girl in my Pilates class so I will look like her."

Psychological Quotient (PQ): Comparing yourself to others is a futile activity because genetic predispositions, dieting history, body types, and biological differences are unique to you, and embracing your autonomy makes you special.

Should Statements: There is a tendency to impose should, could, and must statements onto yourself that becomes self-punitive and create guilt, remorse, and shame. Example: "I must start my diet tomorrow because I hate my body."

Psychological Quotient (PQ): Self-deprecating thoughts do not allow you to grow and evolve as a person and often time these thoughts lead to lack of motivation.

The Hungry Heart Syndrome

"The Hungry Heart Syndrome" describes emotional hunger and may be triggered by specific emotions versus physical hunger. Emotional eating has reached an epidemic proportion, so it is important to understand and prevent the causes of formal eating disorders and obesity. More than five million Americans suffer from eating disorders. Anorexia nervosa, bulimia nervosa, and binge-eating disorder are diseases that affect the mind and body simultaneously. Three percent of adolescent and adult women and one percent of men have anorexia nervosa, bulimia nervosa, or binge-eating disorder. Chronic dieting can be a prelude for an eating disorder or disordered eating. Chronic dieting is the single most predictor for developing a formal eating disorder and girls who diet moderately are 5 times more likely to develop an eating disorder than those who don't diet, and those who diet severely are 18 times more likely. A young woman with anorexia is 12 times more likely to die than other women her age without anorexia. Approximately, 15 percent of young women have substantially disordered eating attitudes and behaviors.

What are the causes and roots of eating disorders? Genetic predispositions such as addictive disorders may be present, and environmental stressors may lead to eating difficulties. In fact, parents, spouses, and loved ones may be the last to learn that someone they love has a formal eating disorder. In a study of children ages eight to ten, approximately half the girls and one third of the boys were dissatisfied with their size. However, most dissatisfied girls wanted to be thinner while about equal numbers of dissatisfied boys wanted to be heavier. Boys wanted to grow into their bodies, whereas girls were more worried about their bodies growing. Recent findings indicate that girls who smoke to suppress their appetite are the highest group of new nicotine addicts. The cigarette industry is aggressively targeting the vulnerability of girls who want to lose weight. Girls who participate in elite competitive sports where body shape and size are a factor (gymnastics, ballet, a cheerleader who is a flyer, and volleyball) are three times more at risk for eating disorders. Boys, who participate in similar sports like wrestling or jockeying are also at increased risk.

Eating disorders are impacting young adults and middle-aged people more than ever. Eating disorders use to be more common among male homosexuals, but our patient census has increased among male heterosexuals. It is not only more prevalent with males in general, but with heterosexual males, often associated with certain careers particularly with actors, journalists, broadcasters, race car drivers, and any career that emphasizes aesthetic qualities or low body weight. Methods of prevention such as addressing mood stability and assessing precipitating factors of emotional eating are important to explore.

Take a moment to see if you or a loved one can identify with the characteristics and symptoms on the spectrum below:

Chronic Dieter or Disordered Eating

Disordered eating and behaviors and attitudes include:

- Binge eating
- Overeating
- Dieting
- Skipping Meals
- Obsessive calorie counting
- Self-esteem based on body shame and weight
- Deprivation due to dieting
- Feeling you cannot normalize your food intake because of fear of weight gain
- Gaining weight after each diet and dramatic weight variances

Formal Eating Disorders

Warning Signals for Binge Eating Disorder (BED):

- Binge episodes
- Eating in secret
- An overwhelming lack of sense of control in regards to eating behaviors
- Eating more rapidly than normal
- Periods of uncontrolled, impulsive or continuous eating
- Eating when not physically hungry
- Repeated episodes of binge eating, which often results in feelings of shame and guilt
- Avoiding social situations, particularly those involving food
- Eating normal quantities in social settings, and bingeing when alone
- Low self-esteem and embarrassment over physical appearance
- Feeling extremely distressed, upset, and anxious during and after a binge episode
- Fear of the disapproval of others
- Self-harm or suicide attempts
- Overly sensitive to references about weight or appearance
- Self-loathing
- Anxiety
- Depression
- Eating in a discrete period of time an amount of food that is larger than most would consume
- Lack of control over your eating and feeling you cannot stop eating
- Eating more rapidly than normal
- Eating until feeling uncomfortably full
- Eating alone because of feeling embarrassed by how much one is eating
- Feeling disgusted with oneself after bingeing

Warning Signs of Anorexia Nervosa

- Preoccupation with body shape, weight and/or appearance
- Intense fear of gaining weight resulting in restricting, fasting, or skipping meals
- Preoccupation with food or food-related activities
- Negative or distorted body image
- Perceiving self to be fat when at a healthy weight/underweight
- Low self-esteem (guilt, self-criticism, worthlessness)
- Rigid thinking
- Amenorrhea (loss of menstrual cycle for a minimum of three consecutive months)
- Cardiac complications
- Feeling out of control
- Mood swings
- Anxiety or depression
- Heightened anxiety around meal times
- Heightened sensitivity to comments or criticism about body shape/weight/appearance/eating/exercise habits
- Suicidal or self-harm thoughts or behaviors
- Constant or repetitive dieting/restrictive or rigid eating patterns
- Excessive or compulsive exercise
- Changes in clothing style
- Obsessive rituals around food
- Changes in food preferences
- Frequent avoidance of eating meals/excused not to eat
- Social withdrawal
- Repetitive or obsessive body checking behaviors
- Deceptive or secretive behavior around food

Warning Signals of Bulimia Nervosa

- Difficulties with activities that involve food
- Loneliness due to self-imposed isolation and a reluctance to develop personal relationships
- Deceptive behaviors relating to food
- Fear of the disapproval of others if the illness becomes known
- Mood swings, changes in personality, emotional outbursts or depression
- Self-harm, substance abuse, or suicide attempts
- Sensitivity to references about weight or appearance
- Guilt, self-disgust, self-loathing
- Anxiety
- Depression
- Frequent trips to the bathroom, especially after eating
- Food avoidance or dieting behavior due to fear of weight gain or to avoid purging
- Fluctuations in weight
- Erratic Behavior
- Binge and purge episodes
- Anxiety
- Depression

Behaviors: Cupcakes and Cakes

Cakes can be baked in a myriad of methods: a two or three tier, an extravagant cake shaped and decorated like a Chanel handbag or unicorn, or a lovely cupcake! You can also choose your favorite flavor, whether it be lemon, chocolate molten, or raspberry. The modern approach to better body esteem also gives one many options by modifying one's behavior. Take a moment to identify if you can relate to the behaviors described below:

Control Freak: No one wants to be a control freak, but often hyper-vigilance develops in regards to controlling food intake because you feel powerless in other areas of your life. Example: "I was blind–sided by my diabetes diagnosis!"

Psychological Quotient (PQ): Become empowered by letting go of the things that you cannot control and not allowing others to control you. If you feel powerless over something, focus on your reaction and how you cope with the challenges presented to you.

Addictive Behaviors: Addictive behaviors such as overuse of technology, alcohol or drug abuse, overeating, overexercising, laxative abuse, smoking cigarettes, and restricting are typically a manifestation of an attempt to sedate emotional distress.

Psychological Quotient (PQ): Identify maladaptive behaviors such as the ones above, and if you are unable to overcome or moderate these behaviors independently, seek professional treatment.

Dying to Be Thin: A relentless pursuit to become thin and a morbid fear of becoming overweight may drive your behaviors to the point that you are willing to compromise your mental and physical health. "I would rather shave off years of my life and stay thin than gain weight."

Psychological Quotient (PQ): Using compensatory behaviors such as restricting or fasting can lead to health complications such as cardiac, osteoporosis, osteopenia, and infertility. Eating disorders have the highest mortality rate of any mental disorder, but we have never lost a patient in our clinics to an eating disorder, and medical monitoring is paramount.

Body Bashing: An extreme dissatisfaction of your body with self-loathing and self-deprecating thoughts. Example: "I weigh myself and do body checks in the mirror several times a day because I hate my body."

Psychological Quotient (PQ): Body image can be improved significantly by increasing your psychological quotient (PQ), nutrition quotient (NQ), exercise quotient (EQ), and fashion quotient (FQ).

Social Alienation: Social isolation is characteristic of emotional eating due to body shame. "I have gained weight since college, and I am not going to attend my class reunion because I feel too fat."

Psychological Quotient (PQ): If you are dissatisfied with your body weight, do not allow it to deter you from enjoying your social life. Read the fashion quotient chapter to learn more ways to improve your body image by becoming your own stylist (#BYOS).

Rigid and Restrictive Behavior: One may become severely restrictive and self-disciplined and avoid all types of indulgences such as food and engage in overexercising as an attempt to offset what is believed to be creating what you are unhappy with. Example: "I have to run every day, or I feel guilty."

Psychological Quotient (PQ): Maintain your exercise regimen but strive for moderation and lighten up on yourself so you can experience a better quality of life.

Your Body as an Instrument: Music Therapy

I encourage you to think outside the box when it comes to boosting your body esteem and mental health. Music is the international language that allows us to transcend to our "happy place." My husband and I toured a musical museum in Belgium on the evolution of all musical instruments that was fascinating. We felt like Tom Hanks in the movie *Big* where we jumped on the keyboard! After touring the museum we both have a greater appreciation for all musical instruments and especially the piano as it evolved from a harpsicord to a concert grand. Instead of obsessing over your body and comparing it to others, try using your body as an instrument because you will have a greater appreciation for your body and be happier. By using your body as an instrument such as taking voice lessons, playing a musical instrument, taking jazz or salsa dancing, joining a choir, or composing lyrics or a musical composition, you may find that you acquire more value for cognitive abilities and your body in general.

According to Harvard Medical School, music engages not only our auditory system, but parts of the brain that are responsible for language, movement, attention, memory, and emotion. Brian Harris, a certified neurologic music therapist at Harvard-affiliated Spaulding Rehabilitation Hospital stated, "There is no other stimulus on earth that simultaneously engages our brains as widely as music does." Furthermore, he reports that this global activation happens whether you are listening to music, playing a musical instrument, or singing in the shower.

Similar to other sensations of pleasure, listening or playing music triggers the release of dopamine, a brain chemical that helps one feel engaged and motivated. Can you imagine dancing without music or going to a party where there is no music? The processing of the sound originates in the brainstem, which also controls heartbeat and respiration. Afterwards, relaxing music may lower blood pressure, heart rate, and breathing. Equally important, music plays a role in reducing pain, stress, and anxiety. According to the American Music Therapy Association, music "provokes responses due to the familiarity, predictability, and feelings of security associated with it." Music takes us back to various times in our life where we can recall where we were and what we were experiencing in that particular moment. The lyrics often resonate with issues we may be experiencing. Music therapy and listening to music has been shown in our clinics to improve body image and psychological health. Listen to your favorite tunes when you feel overwhelmed, stressed, or anxious, and let the music feed your soul.

Psychological Quotient (PQ): Music contributes to heart health and reduces pain, stress, and anxiety.

Tickled Pink: Laughter

Laughter can work wonders on your body image and really is the best medicine! According to Pam Walker, PhD, a psychologist at Cooper Aerobics Center, laughter in a marital system correlates with marital satisfaction and interpersonal attraction. My husband cracks me up with his dry British sense of humor, and our marriage is very flirtatious and playful! Laughter has been shown to reduce stress hormones and tension and induce relaxation. Dr. Walker explains that laughing hard, which has been compared to "internal jogging" results in increase in heart rate, blood pressure, tightened muscles, and respiration. It is similar to a workout because afterwards one experiences muscle relaxation, a calming effect, and respiration and heart rate normalize. Have some belly laughs with friends or if you need a quick laugh, watch talk show host James Corden's YouTube clips of his hilarious carpool karaoke!

Furry Friends: Pet Therapy

I have used pet therapy to build a therapeutic rapport with my patients and especially the ones who have eating disturbances, anxiety, and depression. It works miracles with their mood and body image. They self-disclose more freely as they interact with their dogs and cats because that interaction builds trust in the therapeutic alliance. My clinical observations have been that they become more compliant with their nutrition as they feed their animals and recognize the significance of taking care of themselves and their furry friends. If they are introverted or shy, pets help bring them out of their shell and form a bond with other pet owners. I have had the privilege to work with many equestrians, and equine therapy has also been shown to be clinically effective with patients who have eating disorders or body image issues. More importantly, the unconditional love that animals provide helps with building trust in relationships, overcoming trauma, and developing an overall sense of well-being.

May I introduce you to the newest member of our family, Biggles, our Siamese kitten. He was named after Bigglesworth, a fictional character in British children's books that was a spitfire piolet that my husband loved reading during childhood. Biggles name fits him not because he is "too big," but he arches his back and jumps up in the air and walks sideways every time he is startled. It is his defense mechanism to protect himself from his prey and make himself look larger. It is hilarious! Just like Biggles, pets are known to elevate our mood and help us beat the blues, provide companionship and combat feelings of loneliness, counteract stress hormone levels and reduce anxiety, increase socialization because they are an instant icebreaker, prolong our lifespan, and keep us active. Dogs can actually be your own personal trainer because dog walkers are more likely to stick to a fitness plan than those who walk alone.

How does this work? The theory is that pets boost our oxytocin levels that are also known as the "bonding hormone" or "cuddle chemical," which enhances social skills, decreases blood pressure and heart rate, boosts immune function, and raises tolerance for pain. It also lowers stress, anger, and depression. In fact, pets shower us with so much love it is no surprise they have a big impact on our love organ: the heart. Whether you are going for a walk or cuddling your beloved pet, studies show that this is linked to better cardiovascular health. One ten-year study found that current and former cat owners were 40 percent less likely to suffer a heart attack and 30 percent less likely to die of other cardiovascular diseases. Pets are part of our family, and having these furry friends brings us enormous joy!

The Great Outdoors: Mother Nature

On a delightful note, Mother Nature can actually foster body esteem. A recent study published in the *Journal of Body Image* from researchers at Anglia Ruskin University, Perdana University, and University College London explored the effect that exposure to nature has on people with body insecurities. The results revealed that spending time in nature led to a more positive body image. Put on your sneakers and go for a brisk walk on a nature trail or in a beautiful park and allow this to boost your feelings about yourself and your body. My husband traveled through the Amazon with a guide and had a once-in-a-lifetime experience with nature. Learn to scuba dive or go snorkeling and view the aquatic life, which is tranquil and picturesque. Plan an African safari or stroll through a zoo and observe the sights and sounds of animals or visit a nature preserve near you.

Visit a local garden and stop and smell the roses and enjoy a picnic. My mother grew gorgeous hydrangeas and azaleas in her garden, and she was the happiest when she was gardening. My neighbor Kim is a talented gardener and artist, and her sunny disposition shines through because of her creativity! My husband planted a lovely rose garden for me on Valentine's Day, and I love picking roses and putting them in bud vases or rose bowls. The smell is intoxicating! Years ago I had the honor to chair an event called "Mad Hatters," which is a charity for the Women's Council of Dallas that raises money for the Women's Garden at the arboretum. It was an afternoon filled with hat judging, sipping champagne, a fabulous fashion show, a stroll through the gardens, and an afternoon tea. I was on an emotional high afterwards and not just from the champagne; sharing this experience with my friends and raising money for a charity in the midst of the gardens was exhilarating!

My husband competed in triathlons in Europe and was on the British biathlon team in England, his native country. He taught me how to cross-country ski without using the rifle, of course. While I was learning, all, I could focus on was mastering the technique, the swishing sound of my skies, and the stillness in nature. I skied for five miles my first time, and my commitment to exercise prepared me for the endurance this sport requires. Challenge yourself to use your body as an instrument to pursue an activity you are passionate about versus focusing on becoming thinner or losing weight. You will experience peace of mind, and the results will be more rewarding than you can ever imagine.

Chapter 3
Doing a Number on Yourself

"The scale can only tell you what you weigh, not who you are."
—Steve Maraboli

Ashley Graham, a plus-size model to be the first to grace the pages of *Sports Illustrated* and become a Revlon model, has pioneered the way for many women. During an interview on the *Today* show she stated, "Lipstick has no size!" Our obsession with our body size has become painfully obvious to all, especially in industrialized countries such as America, Europe, and Asia. Our weight, height, and other body measurements are often used to evaluate or judge us, as if there is one standard that is considered the ideal and one that we are all trying to fit. It is not one-size-fits-all when it comes to our body composition. When you allow others to impose, or when you self-impose, a specific standard or paradigm for your body, you are "doing a number on yourself." But, in the truest sense, numerical information is meant to inform. It doesn't have any meaning other than the meanings that are applied to the numbers.

As a psychotherapist, I have seen my patients suffer emotionally, all as a result of a number! By no means am I suggesting that we deny or ignore our body weight as it can serve as a health indicator for our physical and psychological well-being. But the numbers have evolved into something that more often control us or at least stifle our ability to simply enjoy our bodies. There are times that the numbers really count. Eating disorders, cardiac disease, and diabetes are among those numbers that require attention and, often, action. And in conditions such as these, one's need to know their weight because any significant changes can be an important indicator in a larger health issue. But for the rest of us, we often apply too much meaning to the numbers that are part of our physical presentation. Regardless of your weight, the objective is to use the appropriate measurements to assess your physical state and not give the numbers more power than they deserve!

Numbers can be interpreted differently by each person, and it is all about one's perspective. Someone may give value to a specific number whereas someone else may have a completely different viewpoint. Recently, actress Jameela Jamil started a movement called "I Weigh" on an Instagram account on which she posts a spectrum of women sharing their "weight." Jamil's co-star on *The Good Place*, Kristen Bell, posted a photo on her Instagram story saying her weight is "A passion for equality. A partner who challenges me to see all perspectives. An emphasis on giving to others. Two children who keep me laughing. The scar on my stomach that reminds me I did something extraordinary. Friends who double as family. Fiercely fighting for the underdog. A job that fully engages my brain."

Emmy Rossum, an actress and director, is another celebrity who joined the "I Weigh" movement in hopes that other women will view their weight as more than a number on the scale. She wrote on her Instagram story my weight is "Three best friends since kindergarten. Drive. Kindness. Empathy. Jewish and proud. Make friends with strangers. Daughter. 100+ hours of television. The courage it takes every day to overcome PTSD (post-traumatic stress disorder). One happy marriage. Three episodes of television directed."

You, and only you, can give yourself permission to not allow your weight to be a reflection of who you are as a person! You are an amazing human being, and you are much more than the number on the scale! Your capacity to experience life at its fullest is immeasurable. The scale does not reveal your personality traits, measure your intellectual capabilities, level of motivation, or capacity to withstand trials and tribulations. Our code of ethics and level of integrity are not reflected on the scale. More importantly, our self-esteem and body image does not have to be based on what the numbers on the scale say.

Pause for a moment and fill in the blank starting with "I Weigh," omitting any numbers as it relates to your body. I know you are so much more than a number on the scale! Your number known as "your weight" is not meant to be shared with anyone except your healthcare providers, so the next time someone asks you what you weigh, you do not have to disclose this number. Comparing and contrasting your weight sets up unhealthy competition with others. It is a personal matter like your salary or bank account. Your objective, and I strongly encourage you to accept it, is to no longer look to the scale for validation, social conformity, and acceptance.

Porky Pies and Little Lies

Parents often record the height of their children on the wall with their age as they are growing. Children always seem to want to be taller or older. Sometimes they go as far as to tell a lie about their age and say they are older. A lovely English woman once told me she was ninety-one years old, and her son winked and whispered to me that she was actually ninety-six. Cockney language in Britain refers to little lies as "Porky Pies." Women in particular have a tendency to bend the truth (tell porky pies) about their age and weight. As a psychotherapist specializing in body image and eating disorders, I have compassion for our patients who carry so much shame and humiliation related to their weight. It is like carrying the weight of the world on their shoulders. One important aspect of body esteem is to become honest with yourself. Some patient's fear of what the scale will tell as their "real weight" paralyzes their ability and curiosity to know what they weigh so they can monitor their physical health.

Let's explore the underlying reason that the number on the scale has such a profound emotional effect. A study conducted at the University of Central Florida found that nearly half of girls ages three to six worry about being fat, and about one third in this same age range would change a physical attribute such as their weight. It appears that girls in particular are starting to be more obsessional about their weight at a younger age than ever before. As they become older, they are more cognizant of their bodies, and there is a tendency to overestimate or underestimate weight and caloric consumption due to embarrassment and shame. Sadly enough, this number has so much emotional power and control that it actually defines how some of us see ourselves, others, and our quality of life.

I believe that with the proper education we can teach children at an early age to interpret and understand the numbers. Our treatment team collaborates with pediatricians who address the children's and adolescents' weight and normalize the fact that gaining weight and height is part of their physical development. These doctors speak to patients in a compassionate manner, educating them on childhood obesity and eating disorders prevention. This consult and more understanding of what the numbers truly represent make a dramatic difference in how patients receive the message regarding incorporating balanced nutrition, exercise, and, if necessary, counseling about their lifestyles.

The Weight Is Over

Our obsession with weight colors all aspects of our lives. It appears that most of us want to lose weight rapidly, and many find it to be challenging to be patient and make the changes needed to secure sustainable weight loss. If you need to lose weight for medical or psychological reasons, then be patient with yourself and lose it gradually without a trendy diet. I have supported patients who have lost ten pounds to well over one hundred pounds, and those who lose their weight gradually typically maintain their healthy weight range. In the meantime, try to not dwell on your weight, but introduce behavioral changes, and over time, you will experience more satisfaction with your results.

The concepts in this chapter such as the resting metabolic rate test will educate you on how to see numbers in a new way—a way that gives you the advantage. When you overcome the emotions that you experience and understand and embrace your body, your anxiety regarding your weight will reduce over time. As such, the measurements we discuss in this chapter become a powerful tool rather than something to be avoided or dreaded. I welcome you into a world where the following numbers can serve as a guide to a more vibrant and enthusiastic life. Let's explore the numbers that might impact your overall body esteem quotient and how your resting metabolic rate and body composition are unique to only you.

The Number's Game

Supermodel Gigi Hadid decided not to play the "number's game" when critics pounced on some changes in her body as a result of being treated for Hashimoto's disease, a thyroid disorder with symptoms such as fatigue, weight gain, and dry skin. She told her supporters and her critics that at age seventeen, when she returned to modeling, she had not yet been diagnosed and she was criticized for being "too big" for modeling. Hadid states that her heavier appearance was due to inflammation and water retention. Impressively, she states, "I will not further explain the way my body looks, just as anyone with a body type that doesn't suit your beauty expectations shouldn't have to."

I applaud her because she is simply saying that she will no longer play "the numbers game." Posting critical comments on social media in regard to judgements about anyone's weight is mean-spirited. The consequences of irresponsible behavior such as fat shaming is devastating to others and is a behavior that needs to stop! The numbers, whether they be related to age or body proportions, are just numbers. We are the ones who attach meaning and judgment to those numbers. We are the ones who allow those numbers to impact self-esteem or body image. For one moment, imagine taking back every meaning that you've given numbers in choosing how you feel about your body into your own control.

Our obsession with weight may carry over to our age and in the bedroom! Let's examine how our body weight impacts life so you can begin leaving behind your own preoccupation with your weight. *USA Today* reported that the best age for enjoying sex for single women is sixty-six and for men, sixty-four. The study was funded by Dallas-based dating service Match and conducted by Research Now. It revealed that single people over sixty report higher levels of sexual satisfaction. According to the study, a common misconception is that younger people are enjoying sex more. One of the reasons cited for this age was due to the fact that as one ages, they are more "comfortable in their own skin." Likewise, sex and intimacy are often avoided when you are not comfortable with your body or weight. It is heartbreaking to see how our feelings about our body impact a sexual experience that is meant to bring pleasure. Nonetheless, one seems less inhibited while engaging in sex if they are comfortable with their body.

Is the Scale Your Ghost or Your God?

Is the scale your god where you weigh in several times per day or daily, determining how much or what you will eat that day? Perhaps you hide from the scale with fear and have not weighed yourself in ages. Does the scale set the tone for your mood? Do you jump for joy if you have lost a few pounds? Sometimes it may feel that you are on an emotional roller-coaster ride through the ups and downs of life as your body changes. It is important to note that "fat is not a feeling!" In this book, as you address your psychological quotient (PQ), nutrition quotient (NQ), and exercise quotient (EQ), you can begin to make peace with the scale and other forms of measurement for your body.

Body Composition

Body composition is the term used to describe the makeup of the human body through percentages of water, bone, fat, and muscle. This is why two people of the same gender and weight may look entirely different—because they have different body compositions. The body composition measurement is the proportion of fat and fat-free mass in your body. The body composition is often used in clinics as a health indicator as well. One may complete a body composition test at the onset of designing a new physical fitness regimen or when you want to pursue a weight loss program. Many exercise physiologists use it to periodically assess your progress with physical fitness or to provide feedback as you achieve your weight loss goals.

In our clinics, the body composition assessment determines a healthy weight range (HWR) and gauges potential health problems such as amenorrhea, which is the loss of the menstrual cycle for a minimum of three consecutive months. Amenorrhea is a symptom of anorexia nervosa and occurs when the percentage of body fat is low, and it may lead to infertility if not addressed. One's HWR is based on medical stability with normal vital signs and no medical complications such as infertility, bone density (osteoporosis or osteopenia), and cardiac complications. It is not based on some random number that was assigned to you with no empirical evidence to support this. Therefore, your weight is unique to you as an individual and your HWR, along with the calories required to maintain it, are uniquely different than that of others and should be treated as such.

Fat Factoids

If you weigh yourself on a bathroom scale it is important to note the fact that the scale does not assess your body composition. The scale cannot inform you about how much of your total weight is based on water, fat, or muscle. Furthermore, it is completely unrealistic for your body weight to be the same each day, and a variance is not atypical due to changes in bodily functions (ovulation and menstrual cycle, etc.). If you have Thai food for dinner and weigh yourself the next morning your weight may be higher due to the sodium content of the meal you had the night before and the body's retention of water. Diagnoses such as irritable bowel syndrome and endometriosis can cause excessive bloating, causing your weight to widely fluctuate.

Body fat is found under the skin (subcutaneous fat), in muscle mass tissue (intramuscular fat), and around organs (visceral fat). Some of this fat is absolutely necessary for your overall health and is referred to as essential fat. The primary purpose of essential fat is to store food for energy, regulate body hormones, and protect one's internal organs. In contrast, fat-free mass includes bone, water, muscle, organs, and tissues and is commonly referred to as lean mass. These tissues are metabolically active and burn calories for energy and are necessary for your health. Body fat percentage is a measurement of body composition that assesses how much of your weight of your body constitutes fat. Knowing your body fat percentage is a good indication of your health and can be monitored to maintain your health status. Your body fat can serve as a prevention for risk factors for heart disease, stroke, diabetes, and certain types of cancer.

A healthy body fat percentage for a female is approximately 17 percent to 25 percent and for males is about 13 percent to 18 percent. Underweight for women is considered less than 15 percent and obese is more than 32 percent. For males 5 percent is considered underweight and obese is 25 percent or higher. These ranges do vary based on genetics and other biological factors. The normal ranges designated for male and female differ. In my clinical experience, it is not wise to diet with anyone and especially the opposite sex, as males lose weight much faster than females, generally speaking. Your weight is not meant to be a number that you use for competition and comparative analysis because this will often lead to more obsession. As you age, your muscle tissue naturally decreases, and physical activity will foster the prevention of muscle mass loss. Web M.D. contends that physically inactive people can lose as much as 3 percent to 5 percent of muscle mass each decade after age thirty. If you are active, you may still have some muscle mass loss, which varies from person to person.

Lucky Numbers

Do you have a lucky number? Perhaps it is the number you like to use at the derby for winning horse races or the lottery, or perhaps it is your boyfriend's jersey number from football. We do tend to embrace some numbers such as finding a 75 percent off after-Christmas sales at the mall or your favorite boutique. Numbers in regard to our health are useful for prevention and wellness. Kenneth Cooper, MD, MPH, the founder and owner of the Cooper Aerobics Center, advocates "an ounce of prevention is worth a pound of cure." The Cooper Aerobics Center at Cooper Clinic offers annual physical and wellness exams as a form of prevention for positive mental and physical health. People come from all over the world to complete a comprehensive annual preventive physical exam and endorse this philosophy. Prevention and early detection is critical in diagnosing the early stages of health problems such as cancer or cardiac disease.

It is important to know your numbers such as your blood pressure, heart rate, weight, and body composition. There is something reassuring when you hear your mammogram and bone density are within the normal range and your complete blood count (CBC) is in the healthy range. It makes the fact that you have been compliant with exercise (EQ) and balanced nutrition (NQ) a great payoff! If the numbers are not to your liking, such as your triglycerides are elevated, you can use these numbers to empower you to resolve to take on a plan that will improve them! Make it your personal goal to improve your blood work and health. Bear in mind that health-related measurements can improve, and you can change what may be affecting them and make a difference in your test results. Avoiding, dismissing, or minimizing these numbers only prolongs a return to vibrant health, and more complications will eventually emerge if not addressed. That leads to only more anxiety about your health.

The BMI Battle

While popular in some fitness books and with some doctors and other health professional, body mass index (BMI) is not an accurate predictor for one's size, shape, or health! The BMI has become a battlefield for controversy among scientists and professionals! Unlike body composition assessments, the BMI is unpredictable. Historically, it has been considered the standard for measuring the amount of fat in a person's body, and according to the research, it is very controversial. A person's height and weight are the two factors that determine a person's BMI. According to researchers from the University of California, Los Angeles (UCLA), this one-size-fits-all approach may be flawed. Their study, published in the *International Journal of Obesity*, reveals how inaccurate the BMI is in terms of labeling people as overweight or obese, based only on the two measurements of height and weight. It is imperative for doctors and patients to have a more accurate determination for assessing one's healthy weight range since this is such a sensitive subject for most of us. Just for a moment, imagine your doctor deems you overweight or obese when the diagnostic formula to determine this is inaccurate like the BMI.

The BMI bases all its categories only on height and weight and does not take into account a person's bone, muscle, or fat proportions. Did you know that muscle is actually four times as dense as fat tissue? For example, a person with exceptional muscle tone and low fat is more likely to have a higher BMI compared to someone with higher fat and lower muscle tone. Worldwide obesity is a significant problem and is a public health concern, so for this reason alone it is vitally important to use accurate assessments to measure one's healthy weight range.

Nearly half of those whose BMIs labeled them as overweight were actually within their healthy weight range according to alternative body composition measurements. Fifteen percent of those who were classified as obese were also considered healthy. And when the researchers looked at participants classified as healthy, they found 30 percent were actually unhealthy when other health measures were taken into consideration. If the findings were extrapolated to the entire American population, the researchers said as many as fifty-four million people are incorrectly told they're unhealthy.

The BMI was introduced in the mid-1800s. In 1998 the National Institutes of Health approved the BMI as a standard of health measurement, and overnight thirty million Americans moved from a healthy weight category to an overweight one. In my clinical opinion, the BMI has contributed to the increase in the prevalence of eating disorders and obesity due to the fact that it lacks reliability and validity in measuring one's body composition. The BMI is analogous to baking a cake without the precise measurements, and it is possible the cake may not rise or turn out the way you expected it to. Therefore, the BMI needs to be phased out as a standard for body composition and guidelines. It simply is too unreliable and inaccurate.

Similarly, if the BMI scale is eventually deemed as an ineffective tool to measure weight and health risks because of questionable accuracy, there are other avenues for assessment. There are other methods to measure body composition ranging from simple, at-home techniques to complex procedures. One now has other options for a mode of measurement that are more precise and a better indicator of your body composition to choose from, and I encourage you to choose one of the following alternatives:

Tape Measure: Due to the fact that excessive abdominal fat may put you at a greater risk for developing high blood pressure, coronary heart disease, or type 2 diabetes according the Centers for Disease Control and Prevention, one should measure their waistline. The formula is that the circumferences of one's waist should be less than half of your height. Therefore, if you are 5'4" tall (64 inches), your waist circumference should be 32 inches or smaller.

Skin Calipers: This plier-shaped measuring tool can clamp sections of fat from your body such as the chest, arms, abdominals, thighs, and back, and as a result, tally an overall percentage of body fat. One word of caution is that the accuracy of the results is dependent upon the technician measuring you, so it is best to find an exercise physiologist who is experienced with this type of measurement.

Hydrostatic Weighing: This measurement, which is commonly referred to as underwater displacement weighing, is an alternative measurement with a very small margin of error and is the go-to standard for clinical research. It is used at the Cooper Clinic at the Cooper Aerobics Center. You wear your swimsuit for this measurement, which compares a patient's normal body weight outside of the water to their body weight while completely submerged under water. Thus, the physician uses the two numbers in addition to the density of water to calculate an estimate of the patient's body composition.

Dual Energy X-Ray Absorptiometry (DEXA): This particular scan emits high and low energy levels of X-ray beams into the patient, one body part at a time, as they lie on a table. It measures bone mineral density, lean body mass, and fat mass. Technicians can provide an accurate breakdown of the body composition level for each section of the body. And it is without question the most accurate form of body composition measurement.

Adding Up the Numbers

Of course, my purpose is to give you various options of how you might effectively measure your body composition. It is important to be knowledgeable so that you are no longer mislabeling yourself with a faulty measurement. My sincere advice to you is do not beat yourself up over a numbers game. Find reliable measurements that can provide input. My personal endorsement would be to utilize the tape measure, skin calibers, hydrostatic weighing, and DEXA as objective measurements. My hope for you is to not confuse the issue of the "number's game," but to give you reliable information so you can use good judgement and well-researched measurements for accuracy. Using these numbers to influence you to take action or to feel more confident about your health can be extremely helpful. Using any numbers as a source for self-shaming or unhappiness is counterproductive and will keep you entrapped in a mindset that impedes progress and change, if that is what you desire.

The Little Red Dress

Do you own a little black dress? Many of us may have several in our wardrobe for those special occasions! The bigger question is, do you own a red dress or know what it stands for as a woman? In 2004, the American Heart Association (AHA) faced a real challenge with the rise in cardiovascular disease among women. In order to dispel the myths and misunderstandings that heart disease was primarily an older man's disease and to raise awareness of the fact that heart disease and stroke is the number-one killer of women, the AHA created "Go Red for Women" campaign. The purpose was to educate and empower women to take care of their heart health and to become more aware and passionate about this cause. This meaningful movement has inspired others to come together and prevent cardiac disease for women as well as educate them on the warning signals (red flags). Living a heart healthy lifestyle is more important today than ever before!

Approximately 55 percent of women are cognizant of the fact that heart disease is the number-one killer of women. Cardiac disease and strokes cause one in three deaths among women each year. This is more than all of the cancers combined, and these statistics are astounding. The good news is we can change these statistics because 80 percent of cardiac and strokes can be prevented with the proper education, medical care, and being proactive. Many women are unaware of the vital signs that may indicate cardiac complications such as blood pressure or cholesterol readings. Based on current research, a woman who chooses to "Go Red" does as follows: incorporates an exercise routine, has a balanced and nutritious diet, visits her physician for important diagnostic testing, and shares with others the prevention of cardiac disease for women.

The "Go Red for Women" movement is making a difference in how women take care of themselves. Approximately 91 percent of women who go red visited their doctor in the last year, and women who go red are more likely to follow their doctor's advice from taking the proper medications to gaining or losing weight. Women who go red completed the following: 64 percent follow a regular exercise routine; 84 percent talk to and educate their friends and loved ones about heart health, 90 percent have their blood pressure checked annually, and 75 percent had their cholesterol checked in the last year. These are numbers one can get behind and use to support their heart health! Prevention and wellness is the name of the game when it comes to women and cardiac disease. But what if some women are fearful of going to their doctor due to being "fat shamed" about their weight?

Joan Chrisler, PhD, a professor of psychology at Connecticut College, stated during her presentation on "Weapons of Mass Distraction—Confronting Sizeism" the following: "Disrespectful treatment and medical fat shaming, in an attempt to motivate people to change their behavior, is stressful and can cause patients to delay health care seeking or avoid interacting with their providers." If your physician or cardiologist or any doctor for that matter, is not speaking to you in a kind and respectful manner regarding your health and weight, then find a new doctor. There are many doctors who are tactful and empathic in their delivery of the message. It is imperative that you not avoid taking care of your physical and mental health because someone is shaming you, especially your doctor and other health professionals.

Building body esteem absolutely includes taking care of your physical health. Bear in mind that when someone gains weight, it may not be for behavioral reasons only. If one gains weight due to lack of exercise or poor nutrition, it is important to take responsibility for your behavior and implement a lifestyle change. However, as we have established, weight gain can be due to hormonal imbalances, menopause, medical conditions (i.e., fibromyalgia), or genetic predispositions. I strongly recommend that you find quality healthcare providers who care about your health as reflected in their bedside manner. Do not be afraid to assert yourself, and do your homework when it comes to your healthcare.

Rev Up Your Engine: Resting Metabolic Rate

Do you love sports cars or enjoy putting your hair in a ponytail and driving a convertible? Your metabolism is somewhat similar to a car in that it has to keep the engine running well. The resting metabolic rate (RMR) is the rate at which the body uses energy while at rest to keep body functioning such as breathing and keeping warm (thermogenesis), cellular growth, and cellular maintenance. RMR is a physiological marker used to objectively measure your metabolism, which is individualized to only you. In the same way that your DNA cannot be replicated, your metabolism represents your individualized body physiology. Your body type, resting metabolic weight, and genetic predispositions are all unique, so comparing your body to anyone else's is counterproductive. Your body will not respond in the same manner or with identical outcomes to someone else, even a sibling or parent, with regard to diet and exercise.

Therefore, make a commitment to yourself that you will no longer compare apples to artichokes when it comes to comparing diets, clothing size, and exercise regimens with others. This is no different that wishing you had blue eyes instead of brown ones! Body comparisons regarding caloric consumption, exercise, and weight lead to frustration and discouragement. For example, each of our patients has a different nutrition program that is unique to their metabolism. It is not a one size fits all when it comes to your metabolic rate. Put effort into learning how to "rev up your engine!" In other words, focus on maintaining or even increasing your metabolic rate and avoid behaviors that slow down your metabolism. After all, there is only one you! Dare to be you!

Resting Metabolic Rate

Resting metabolic rate (RMR) is defined as the energy expended while resting and accounts for the largest component of total energy expenditure in humans (50 to 65 percent). The RMR is dependent on oxygen consumption, in that for every liter of oxygen consumed 4.8 calories are burned. Lean body mass has a higher rate of oxygen consumption than does fat. Therefore, individual RMR varies depending on body composition.

Your RMR is the sum of all vital processes in your body by which energy and nutrients from food are made available to use in your body. Your RMR is the amount of energy needed to keep all your vital processes functioning. This does not include activity, exercise, digestion, or absorption. Your RMR is the amount of energy you would need if you were to stay in bed all day long and just rest; it accounts for 70 to 85 percent of the calories you burn in a day. RMR test results differ from one person to the next based on age, gender, body composition, activity level, and genetic predispositions.

Rebounding

If you are worried that you have permanently lowered your RMR, I have great news for you! It can rebound back to its normal level with patience and behavioral changes. The purpose is to help protect a genetically determined weight and energy balance. The *American Journal of Clinical Nutrition* defines chronic dieting syndrome as "going on and off of calorie restricting for over two years" as well as being "obsessed with weight and size." Chronic dieting has become a syndrome since it has become commonplace to be on some diet whether it be paleo, keto, low carbohydrate, or low fat. This study reported that 85 percent of women will go on a diet in their lifetime, and many will continue various dieting techniques for up to seventeen years! It is not uncommon for dieters to make approximately four to five attempts at dieting per year. Men pursue chronic dieting as well, but in my clinical experience it is more common with females.

In addition, chronic dieting camouflages the road to health and wellness and can be deceptive. In reality, chronic dieting sets you up to be nutritionally deficient, slows down the metabolism, leads to high blood pressure, is often associated with depression and anxiety, and does a number on your psyche. You may feel like a failure since chronic dieting does not have positive long-term effects. So why do you suppose that we keep signing up for the newest fad in dieting? The following are the reasons that the research shows how we become chronic dieters:

- Chronic dieting is enticing in that it gives one the false illusion that one has complete control over their body, food, and lifestyle.
- There are moments of some success which is similar to intermittent negative behavior reinforcement.
- It reinforces that one is vigilant and virtuous (i.e., good girls don't eat chocolate).

- It sets up a vicious cycle of feeling defeated because chronic diets do not work!
- It is alluring in that if one believes if they continue to be compliant with each new diet, it might work.

A Harvard study reported that the best diet is one that we can maintain for life and that it only be one aspect of our healthy lifestyle. You are not a failure! The diets are the ones that are failing you! I challenge you to turn over a new leaf because in order to build body esteem, you must no longer pursue chronic dieting. The time is now to normalize eating (*NQ*). After all, chronic dieting is often a precipitating factor for obesity and eating disorder. You will experience a better quality of life if you commit to not being a chronic dieter!

If you have been a chronic dieter or suffered from a formal eating disorder, there is hope and success in improving your RMR. The total amount of calories you burn in a day is equal to your RMR, daily activity, and exercise. Moreover, there are many factors that impact your metabolism, such as restricting food intake and experiencing significant weight loss, as is the case of anorexia nervosa. As one becomes weight restored and gradually increases one's metabolism, this serves as protection from a significant weight gain. If you have been using compensatory behaviors such as bingeing and purging or overexercising, in the case of bulimia nervosa, and not replenishing your body with adequate calories, your RMR has probably decreased but can be reset.

Set Point Theory

It is believed by an increasing number of scientists that the brain and body automatically set the body's weight range. In some respects, one can take solace in the fact that once you reach your healthy weight range (HWR), it may be easier to maintain this with adequate nutrition and exercise. Maladaptive or compensatory behaviors such as restricting, bingeing and purging, laxative abuse, diuretics, or overexercising are not effective for long-term weight management. There appears to be a control system built into humans by which the body weight range is programed to function optimally. In essence, this phenomenon has commonly been referred to as the "set point theory," and it is responsible for the body to maintain that optimal weight range.

Scientists have discovered that a prune-shape cluster of nerves on the underside of the brain called the hypothalamus may be responsible for controlling appetite. The lateral part of the hypothalamus contains the aptly named weight regulating mechanism that is thought to reduce or increase the body's desire to eat. An example of how the hypothalamus works differently can be illustrated with our Siamese cats named Brahms and Liszt. Since my husband is British and I play classical piano, we named our cats using cockney language. In England, the saying goes "Brahms and Liszt got pissed," which means that they got drunk at the pub! Our American friends think we named them after the great composers, and our English friends laugh and say you have two Siamese alcoholics. Brahms does not have a regulated hypothalamus since he craves food all of the time and will eat as much as possible. Liszt will eat small amounts and often not finish his food in one setting but will return for more food later. Significant progress is made with patients via psychiatric consult for medication regimen, nutrition, psychotherapy, and implementing the hunger rating scale to improve the functioning of the hypothalamus and regulate appetite control.

As humans we all have a certain body fat percentage, and this particular fat content has been established by the set point theory. The weight regulating mechanism will then strive to maintain the determined constant. The set point may stay the same for a considerable amount of time even though the individual may be overfeeding or starving. This is achieved by adjusting a number of physiological functions such as the resting metabolic rate. An analogy would be a house thermostat that is set at a room temperature of 75 degrees and the ambient temperature becomes colder. The thermostat will increase the heat to keep the temperature constant. Similarly, if an individual decreases caloric levels, to prevent starving to death the weight regulating mechanism will kick on a series of physiological functions to try to keep the body weight at the set point. In conclusion, when the body is threatened by starvation (weight loss), it is thought that the control center defends the set point weight by increasing the appetite.

Fat Cell Theory

The fat cell theory is another aspect of the numbers game that can inform you about weight fluctuations throughout the life cycle. Many people fear gaining weight. Perhaps they see others or family members gain weight, and they have anxiety that this will happen to them. Many are constantly assessing and comparing their size against others their age or in their social group or even against celebrities.

The truth is, we all have fat cells. Even though some are convinced that we are gaining fat cells as we age, fat cells are produced during the following times in one's lifespan: (1) last trimester of prenatal life up to the first year of infancy, (2) between the ages of four and seven, (3) during the years between nine and thirteen, and (4) when the body becomes obese, more fat cells are produced to contain that excess fat.

For girls, fat cells will increase during puberty due to the fact that the body is preparing essential fat that is required for females to be fertile later in life. Most girls gain weight prior to starting their first menstrual cycle and typically lose this as they grow taller. It is imperative to reassure females of this age that this is a natural physiological stage of their development and avoid fat shaming. Pediatricians who show compassion and educate patients on this matter can help reduce any fear or anxiety for their patients. The good news is that if you are not genetically predisposed to a significant weight gain, you are less likely to gain weight unless it is due to your behavior (i.e., overeating and lack of exercise). Having knowledge on the fat cell production will hopefully inspire you to not be as anxious about the possibility of weight gain.

Like Mother, Like Daughter

When it comes to positive body image and self-esteem, mothers have a significant impact on their daughters. It is not uncommon for daughters to compare their eating habits, body type, and body image issues with their mothers and look to them as a model for how their body might take shape. The research shows that it is common for someone who has an eating disorder to compare themselves to first-degree biological relatives. Educating them on the simple fact that your nutritional needs are different due to the fact that your metabolism slows down as you age and that we should avoid making comparisons. None of us are perfect, but if you observe signs of low self-esteem and body image issues with your daughter, approach her with compassion and kindness without being critical of her body. Many mothers have made derogatory comments about their own body in front of their children during swimsuit season, setting an expectation for their children and assigning value to similar ideals. Do not induce guilt upon yourself and, by proxy, your children. If you engage in negative body talk with your daughters about yourself, others, or have been critical of your daughter's body, take responsibility and apologize and vow to not do this in the future. Educate them on the techniques in this book so they too can have beautiful body esteem.

If you see signs of a formal eating disorder, act immediately and seek out nutrition counseling and psychotherapy from a licensed dietitian and mental health professional who has expertise in eating disorders. I have worked with many patients who had disordered eating habits but were able to avoid an eating disorder with some education and preventive techniques. Modeling behavior from both parents where you do not pursue restrictive weight loss diets or talk about dieting, weight loss, or exercise frequently is key. It is interesting to note that during my family assessment for an eating disorder, typically one or more family members are chronic dieters and are at that time, on a popular diet. Perhaps this causes more obsession with children because they report they feel they need to be on a diet too. Normalize your eating habits as a family and implement nutritious meals and exercise. Forgive yourself and remember that excessive guilt is a symptom of depression, so move forward. Simply pull yourself up by your bra straps, as we say in Texas, and learn from your past mistakes.

In addition, the most common mistakes that parents make are as follows: introducing dieting techniques to your children at an early age and treating female children differently from males. For example, the girls are served a turkey sandwich and fruit for lunch and the boys are served peanut butter and jelly and chips. Perhaps this sends a message that the girls cannot trust their judgement when it comes to food choices or that they cannot learn the art of mindful eating. Most children are naturally intuitive eaters, and when one controls their food intake, it does not allow the children to use this genetically predisposed technique.

Jeanetics Factors

There is nothing more pleasing than finding the right pair of jeans! Imagine pulling on your favorite jeans that are soft and comfortable and going for a Saturday morning coffee with man's best friend. The jeans hug you in all of the right places, and best of all, they flatter your figure. We all love our blue jeans and different types of jeans fit or flatter a variety of body types. The fashion quotient chapter (𝓕𝑄) will help you enlist the techniques of fashion and style to enhance your appearance, using your body to dictate your best look. Just as with weight, don't play the numbers game with clothing sizes. We give this number too much emotional control, especially when it comes to jeans and swimsuit sizes. Designers cut the styles differently, and for this reason it is important to "not do a number on yourself" when it comes to your wardrobe.

Genetic predispositions play an important role when it comes to our body size, weight, and body types, and I often refer to this as jeanetic factors. Therefore, comparing your clothing size to your mother or sister or friends is unrealistic, and exchanging clothes is not warranted. Historically, I have noticed that when girls and women exchange clothes, it sets them up to obsess about clothing sizes and comparing body types. Even if you are both a size 10, different articles of clothing may fit you each differently due to body composition. Be loyal to yourself and wear your own clothing, and do not let the numbers dictate how your clothes fit you!

Score Card

We are surrounded with score cards in life, whether it be a game such as a tennis match, bank account, or your complete blood work for your health status. These scores or numbers do not dictate our future, but instead give us the opportunity to change it and see the numbers through a new lens. In conclusion, the "numbers game" can be viewed as simply numbers, statistics, or accurate forms of measurements. The challenge for all of us is to use our numbers in a productive manner that boost our body esteem quotient (𝓑𝓔𝑄). If you are not happy with some of your numbers (i.e., percentage of body fat or RMR), do not dwell on them but implement behavioral changes. Don't just talk about making changes. None of these numbers are written in stone and most often can be improved over time. If your blood glucose levels are elevated and you are genetically predisposed to diabetes, increase your exercise and educate yourself on preventive techniques. Take control of your health status, heed the warning signals, and be proactive so you can avoid developing diabetes. If you have been a dieter, obese, or had a formal eating disorder, challenge yourself to overcome this and consider getting professional help. Don't interpret your need for help as a weakness or flaw. See it as the most powerful thing you can do for yourself because you are investing in yourself! The other chapters will provide you with more tools on coping with the nutrition quotient (NQ), exercise quotient (EQ), psychological quotient (PQ), and fashion quotient (FQ), which will in turn improve how you see the numbers!

Chapter 4
Exercise: Move It!

"Time is a dressmaker specializing in alterations."
—Faith Baldwin

For years, Nike has used the slogan "Just Do It" to motivate people to exercise. When it comes to exercise, many of us have good intentions to pursue and maintain an exercise regimen. More often than not, the real challenge is not commencing an exercise program but staying committed to and motivated about one. A report from the World Health Organization found that people in the UK were among the least active in the world, with 32 percent of men and 40 percent of women reporting inactivity. In the meantime, obesity is adding to the chronic long-term diseases cited in the Public Health England's analysis, which shows women in the UK are dying earlier than in most European countries.

According to Michelle Segar, the director of the University of Michigan's Sport, Health and Activity Research and Policy Center, the reasons for beginning to exercise are fundamental to whether we will keep it up! She contends that too often "society promotes exercise and fitness by hooking into short-term motivation: guilt and shame." She reported that some younger people will go to the gym more if the rationale is appearance-based, but after our early twenties this is not what motivates us, nor do vague goals such as wanting to lose weight. However, in her book entitled *No Sweat: How the Simple Science of Motivation Can Bring You a Lifetime of Fitness,* she says we will be victorious if we focus on immediate positive feelings such as stress reduction. She states, "The only way we are going to prioritize time to exercise is if it is going to deliver some kind of benefit that is truly compelling and valuable to our daily life."

Jazz it Up: Exercise and Variety

I love the musical and movie *Chicago,* and one of my favorite tunes from it is "All That Jazz," but sometimes we are not so jazzed to exercise! The good news is you do not have to love working out in order to be compliant with an exercise routine. In fact, one of the essential components to maintain an exercise program is enjoying the benefits of exercise for your psychological and physical health. Quite honestly, my favorite part of exercising is when it is over! I experience the psychological benefits of less anxiety and stress, and I realize it was all worth it and enjoy a glass of French chardonnay!

Exercise does not have to be boring and mundane, torturous or even unpleasant. In fact, changing things up may keep you more committed to your exercise routine. Begin to think of all movement as exercise and suddenly your choices expand. Think of walking, volleyball, or ice skating. Jennifer Aniston told Women's Health, "I have a lot of favorite workouts. Variety is the key for me." She reportedly keeps it interesting by varying the cardio machines she uses (bike, treadmill, and elliptical) and completing interval training between low and vigorous intensities. Go ahead and jazz up your workout to avoid being bored to tears!

My piano teacher lives in Colorado and is eighty-one years old and snowshoes and hikes frequently to train for vigorous mountain hikes like Kilimanjaro! She is a great role model in that she is physically fit and a virtuoso pianist—a balance of sitting and moving in her life! She values brain health and physical fitness, both of which show in her adventurous spirit, passion for playing the piano, and hiking! She once told me that one of her young students said, "You look like a teenager from the back." She roared with laughter. She is an incredibly confident and talented teacher, and she seems ageless! Exercise improves your quality of life throughout your lifespan, and your exercise quotient ($\mathcal{E}Q$) is an important factor that will enhance your overall body esteem quotient ($\mathcal{BE}Q$).

Web MD cites six reasons why people do not exercise: fatigue, no time, previous trials of exercise, parental responsibilities, boredom, and don't enjoy movement. In actuality, I am not wild about exercise, but I am married to an exercise physiologist and a former member of the British biathlon and triathlon teams. He has seen throughout his career how important it is to build both value and variety in exercise so you will stay motivated and committed. You do not have to be an athlete to benefit from swimming, walking, or running and as long as you are active, you will receive the therapeutic effects.

$\mathcal{E}Q$: Jumpstart your exercise regimen and make a list of the benefits that you would like to achieve, such as have better body image, overcome insomnia, and improve your endurance, flexibility, and strength via physical fitness.

Sharp as a Razor: Brain Health and Exercise

Do you ever feel like you have pushed the pause button on your memory? I love to learn, and my husband and I share a strong intellectual curiosity! He has acquired a wealth of knowledge in European literature, world affairs, photography, sports, travel, and philosophy. There is nothing sexier than a man who engages in thought-provoking conversation! The beauty of lifelong learning is that you are not restricted to a syllabus or specific subject matter, and you may choose what interests you! A growing body of research reveals that exercise contributes to brain health and enhances brain functioning. In my clinical opinion, anytime you can engage in and maintain physical activity, it promotes body positivity and improves cognitive functioning.

Exercise increases your heart rate, which pumps more oxygen to the brain and releases a plethora of hormones that provide a nourishing environment for the growth of brain cells, analogous to a lush garden that produces healthy fruits and vegetables. You have probably heard of "runner's high," which acts as a mood elevator and decreases stress hormones. A study in Stockholm found that the antidepressant effect of running was also associated with more cell growth in the hippocampus, the area of the brain responsible for learning and memory. What is the allure of a mud run? A mud run is a mixture of whimsical fun and physical exertion where a good bit of the activity takes place in the mud; it is the perfect event for someone who is ready to make a positive change but needs a cloak to do it under. If you are not afraid of getting down and dirty, then train for a mud run and bond with new mud buds and boost your growth of brain cells!

If getting muddy is not your style, sign up for one of the races with charitable motives to really make your participation count, and you will feel good about supporting a great cause. You may choose from Zombie Run, Color Run, Turkey Trot, Undie Run (I think I will skip the underwear run!), Jingle Bell Run, Bun Run (afterwards you receive a hot cross bun), or a photo op with Mickey Mouse. Today's most amazing themed races feature insane obstacles, over-the-top costumes, and an outrageous supply of tasty treats. The best part is that these wild and crazy events get the body, mind, and spirit off to the races. There is truly something for everyone, including a Hot Chocolate Race for chocoholics who receive a gift bag of Ghirardelli chocolates. If you want a real adventure, pursue the Galapagos Marathon since it is the only race in the world where you'll see giant tortoises and sea lions along the way and experience a lovely human connection at this small, intimate event on San Cristobal Island. I think I will add this one to my bucket list.

Do It with Style

Different exercise styles are associated with brain functioning during and after working out. For years dance therapy and yoga have been used as an adjunct treatment for positive body image. Ballroom dancing utilizes both mental and physical requirements and has a significant impact on cognitive functioning over just exercising or completing a mental task by itself. Many years ago, I persuaded my husband to take ballroom dance lessons. Initially our teacher recommended that we dance in our slippers because we kept stepping on each other's toes. We were both amazed at the mental and physical exertion required to master various dances like the tango, foxtrot and East Coast swing. The good news is we eventually advanced to purchasing dance shoes!

The best exercises are the ones that integrate different parts of the brain, such as coordination, rhythm, and strategy. My husband loves adventure sports: rock climbing, paragliding, windsurfing, and kayaking, and all of them foster brain health. If you are not into dancing (i.e., salsa, hip hop, jazz, or ballet) or adventure sports, there are other types of strategic sports that meet the requirement of stimulating different parts of the brain such as baseball, basketball, racquetball, and tennis. The objective is to engage your cognitive abilities simultaneously as you are moving. Formulate concepts for designing a business plan, or listen to music you are learning to master on your musical instrument (guitar, piano, or violin) as you go for a walk or run. Allow your creative temperament to kick in as I did while exercising and developing concepts for this book! Your imagination can take you places that you have never dreamt of, and all the while you are improving your brain functioning and physical fitness! Of course, always stay alert to your surroundings and keep personal safety at the forefront of any plan!

All in all, choosing physical exercises that improve brain health can be good for your heart as well as your brain. In addition, aerobic exercise improves brain function and acts as a first-aid kit to damaged brain cells. Studies show if you exercise in the morning, you will receive the following benefits: increased brain activity, improved stress management, retention of new information or data, and better reaction to complex situations. A circuit of weights will increase your heart rate and allow you to continuously focus and redirect your attention for each weight machine. If you find yourself mentally fatigued, do a few jumping jacks or jump rope to reactivate your ability to focus and concentrate. As you are on the elliptical ask your virtual assistant such as Alexa or Cortana the question of the day or learn new factoids.

Exercise Quotient (EQ): Exercise that requires cognitive functioning and physical exertion promotes brain health and physical fitness.

The Two-fers

My philosophy is to "find joy in the journey!" If we allow ourselves to explore the endless possibilities, we may be able to find the secondary gain (Nancy Komen's walk for breast cancer prevention) or positive reinforcement (a chai tea latte or iced coffee) after our exercise regimen.

Multi-tasking can sometimes be a challenge, but it may be easier if you are achieving other objectives simultaneously along with your physical activity. If you are planning to snow ski over the holiday season, improve your level of fitness to sustain and endure the sport. Practice roller skiing or working out on a cross country ski machine, and you will be soaring down the slopes or skiing the beautiful countryside. If you love music or books on tape, plug one in as you go for a walk in your neighborhood. Once you attend the next concert you will be familiar with the music and prepared for the book club meeting. Learn a foreign language such as French, German, or Spanish as you use the elliptical. Binge watch your favorite series or watch a good thriller while you are on the treadmill or the rowing machine, and time will fly! Satisfy your competitive nature while competing with others via a Peloton.

If you love playing golf, walk the course in lieu of riding in the golf cart as you close the next business deal. If you adore being outdoors, take your dog to play Frisbee in the park, and if you're single, you may just meet another dog lover! If you are a social butterfly, join a Pilates class and make new friends. If you are a new mother experiencing postpartum depression and it is difficult to find time to exercise, take your baby for a long stroll or join a stroller strides exercise class for new moms. Book a date with your friend you have not seen in ages to exercise together or schedule appointments in advance with a personal trainer to mark this off your calendar. Increasing numbers of businesses now have a gym, so plan a business discussion over a workout or brisk walk around a nearby track. If you are in walking distance, walk or bike to and from work. It will jumpstart your preparation for a productive day and help you unwind and destress after a busy one. Try the latest local fun exercise such as goat yoga or simulated surfing. If you are near water, think of rowing, paddle boarding, or kayaking. Novelty exercise experiences are memorable, and as such, stimulate a different area of the brain. Plus, they are fun!

Personality traits have a strong correlation with sports preferences. They play a significant role as to whether you will commit and excel in a particular physical activity. Don't leave participation up to willpower and scheduling alone. Tap into your known resource of personality traits to find a good match in sports and activities. In the same way that you have deal breakers for relationships and business dealings, you likely have deal breakers in physical activities as well. In our clinics, we often use several personality test results as a roadmap to psychological health, but to also help guide our patients in their exercise regimen. The Myers-Briggs personality test which is used in business and clinics identifies if one is introverted or extroverted. One can be a bit of both, but you may want to allow your personality traits to guide you to the exercise that fits your personality. Introverted people tend to be more subdued, quiet and thoughtful whereas extroverts are more gregarious, loud, and excitable. Why is this so important? If you are an introvert and not an athlete and have no desire to engage in team sports, you might pursue a private or group yoga class which is more in keeping with your personality traits and comfort zone.

According to research the following are guidelines for introverts: concentration, precision, self-motivation, intricate skills, low arousal levels, and individual performances (i.e., archery, cycling, running or golf). Conversely, extroverts prefer sports which are: exciting, team sports, fast paced, high arousal levels, and low concentration (i.e., rugby, boxing, dancing, tap dancing or baton twirling). Yes, I was a majorette and drum major and loved it due to my gregarious personality and passion for music! I discovered recently that batons now come in bright colors and I just had to purchase a hot pink one!

EQ: Identify if you are an extrovert or introvert or a mixture of both and correlate your exercise regimen with a sport or routine that matches your personality traits.

On the Road Again: Exercise and Travel

Have you heard about Singapore's Changi Airport which was voted number one in the world? I would love to go back to Singapore just to check out the amenities: a free movie theater, a butterfly garden, a rooftop swimming pool, and 24-hour spas are just a few. Traveling for business or pleasure can sometimes be exhausting and especially if you are going through different time zones or your flight is delayed or canceled. Utilize the time in the airport to go for a walk and treat yourself to a chair massage. If you are a frequent traveler, pack your jump rope or stay at hotels that have a fitness room. One of our dearest friends is a successful entrepreneur that we admire and respect enormously and he still travels for business at the age of 83. He never misses his swimming or biking workouts while he is traveling, and we go on vacation with him and his lovely wife and many people mistakenly think he is the same age as my husband!

My husband, Philip and I mastered the Viennese waltz and planned a trip to the musical triangle: Prague, Budapest, and Vienna. The music and anticipation of planning and achieving our goal was unforgettable! On your next holiday naturally plan to incorporate physical activity into your trip such as sightseeing via biking or walking. Take a road trip where hiking and walking and having a picnic are a part of your holiday. Go scuba diving, snorkeling, swimming, jogging, or horseback riding on the beach. Plan to do a walking or bike tour in any city you visit.

The questions below can help to connect you with your thoughts and attitudes toward exercise as an effort to assess you Exercise Quotient (EQ).

Exercise Quotient (EQ) Assessment

1. What are the 4 most important types of exercise?
   a. Talking on your cell, cycling, biking, swimming
   b. Sedentary, walking, sleeping, stretching
   c. Rope jumping, running, resting, eating
   d. Strengthening, stretching, balance, and aerobic

2. Aerobic exercise helps with which of the following?
   a. Relax blood vessel walls and lowers blood pressure
   b. Burns body fat and lowers blood sugar levels
   c. Increases mood and improves body image
   d. All of the above

3. Aerobic exercise reduces
   a. Risk of cardiac disease and colon and breast cancer
   b. Stroke and type 2 diabetes
   c. Depression and anxiety
   d. All of the above

4. The resting metabolic rate test measures
    a. Measures your percentage of body fat
    b. Balances your hormones
    c. Is not useful in designing an exercise regimen
    d. Measures precisely how many calories one needs at rest ★

5. Stretching is an important part of your exercise because it
    a. Feels good and helps you maintain flexibility
    b. Prevents you from pulling a muscle
    c. Burns up more calories
    d. All of the above

6. As we age we
    a. Lose muscle mass
    b. Should not exercise as much
    c. Only do aerobic exercise
    d. Use strength training to become a body builder

7. Why are some people more committed to exercise?
    a. They see the value in it
    b. They do the same exercise routine such as walking
    c. They only want to lose weight
    d. They feel guilty if they do not workout

8. The studies show that exercise is beneficial for
    a. Physical health
    b. Mental health
    c. Longevity
    d. All of the above

9. After age 60 one should incorporate more
    a. Aerobic exercise
    b. Less exercise in general
    c. More strength training
    d. Less strength training

10. The Fitnessgram is
    a. Used for the geriatric population
    b. Used for mothers after giving birth
    c. Used in the school system for children and adolescents
    d. Used only for adults

11. Does exercise help one
    a. Become more physically fit
    b. Improve genetic and biological predispositions
    c. Lose weight
    d. Both A and C

12. No pain, no gain
    a. Is essential to an exercise program
    b. Is an exercise myth
    c. Means you are losing weight
    d. Burns excessive amounts of carbohydrates

13. The body burns in the following order during exercise
    a. Carbohydrates, fat and protein
    b. Protein, fat, and carbohydrates
    c. Stress, dairy, protein
    d. no special order

14. Essential fat is more prevalent in
    a. Women and Men
    b. Women
    c. Boys and Men
    d. Girls and Boys

15. Exercise has the following psychological benefits
    a. reduces anxiety and depressive symptoms
    b. Improves body image and symptoms of ADHD and PTSD
    c. Helps manage stress
    d. All of the above

Overcoming the Moody Blues:
Exercise and Depression

Jumpstarting an exercise program may conjure up some negative emotions initially because you may feel uncomfortable about your body. Perhaps you feel like it is too late, or too much of a bother, or that your body has changed too much, and you are self-conscious about how you look now. You might be putting up barriers and blockages telling yourself that you are too busy, or you don't have the right shoes or clothes. Please accept this truth: You are stronger than you understand, and I have confidence in your ability to master this. Once you commence with exercise whether you have exercised in the past and stopped for some reason or never exercised, the benefits of exercise will overcome these emotions. It will become another health habit like staying well hydrated or taking your vitamins.

The psychological benefits are numerous: improved mood, reduced anxiety, less stress, and minimization of depressive symptoms. One major benefit of exercise is the prevention and improvement in symptoms of depression such as increase in libido. Exercise also helps with seasonal affective disorder (SAD) which is more common in women and the lack of ultraviolet light is a contributing factor. I have seen remarkable results in our patient population with exercise used as part of their treatment plan for overcoming the moody blues. No more holiday blues or reoccurrences of depression! More specifically, depression is often treated with psychotherapy and a psychiatric consult that includes a medication regimen; however according to the Cooper Institute, exercise has been shown to be a great adjunct in the prevention and treatment of depression. Your psychological quotient (PQ) will improve significantly with an exercise prescription.

The Cooper Institute's studies have found that regular exercise can help improve mental health. It can help manage the symptoms of depression, as well as anxiety and low self-esteem. Likewise, regular exercise can also help in overcoming addictions and controlling weight. Unlike some treatment plans for depression, exercise does not have to be a strict regimen. Any type of exercise is beneficial for mental and physical health, so take part in activities you enjoy! Insomnia or sleeping too much are symptoms of depression. If you want to sleep like a baby, I have found with myself and patients that exercise is the best natural sedative for a good night's sleep.

Exercise Quotient (EQ): Exercise improves mental health such as depression, stress, self-esteem, anxiety, body image and addictive disorders.

The Cooper Institute has performed extensive research from its database of more than 100,000 at Cooper Aerobics Center to determine the impact of exercise on the symptoms of depression and anxiety. The research reveals that exercise can be effective in treating and preventing mild to moderate depression, and that effectiveness grows stronger the more you exercise. "People who were fitter had less depressive symptoms and better emotional well-being," says Laura DeFina, MD, Medical Director of Research at The Cooper Institute.

"Additional research showed that people who were fitter over time develop less depression as well." Researchers learned that the more exercise, the better. People who habitually exercise showed the best results. Not only can exercise immediately help to improve symptoms of depression and feelings of anxiety, but it also appears to offer long-term effects. "Exercise can be helpful in treating depression symptoms along with medication," says Dr. DeFina. It can also be beneficial if medicines have not worked completely by improving people's perception of quality of life. "For people who are not depressed, our literature has suggested that they have greater emotional well-being from being fit or fitter." Therefore, if you want to improve your exercise quotient and your psychological quotient, a regular exercise routine does both.

Overcoming Life's Challenges: Exercise and Mental Health

It is well documented in the literature that regular exercise can improve your mental health, but it can also have a profound positive effect in treating Attention Deficit Disorder with Hyperactivity (ADHD) and Post-Traumatic Stress Disorder (PTSD). Exercising regularly is one of the easiest and most effective ways to reduce the symptoms of ADHD and improve concentration, motivation, memory, and mood. Physical activity immediately boosts the brain's dopamine, norepinephrine, and serotonin levels—all of which affect focus and attention. In regard to post traumatic stress disorder where one experiences trauma like date rape, sexual abuse, sexual misconduct or harassment, exercise can be incredibly therapeutic on your road to recovery.

Depression, Generalized Anxiety Disorder, ADHD, and Obsessive-Compulsive Disorder are all comorbid with formal eating disorders and I have noted that exercise decreases symptoms with these diagnoses. You do not have to be a fitness fanatic to enjoy the benefits. Research indicates that modest amounts of exercise can make a difference and elevate one's mood. Regardless of your age or level of fitness, it will enhance your body image and improve your overall mental health. Other mental health benefits include: less lethargic, increased energy, decrease in anxiety attacks and anxiety, improved memory recall and concentration, and obsessive-compulsive tendencies are reduced.

Exercise Quotient (EQ): Physical activity immediately boosts the brain's dopamine, norepinephrine, and serotonin levels which help improve concentration and exercise can be a mood elevator.

Worry Warts: Exercise and Anxiety

Chronic worry and anxiety can be genetically predisposed, but can be managed with exercise, psychotherapy, and medication regimen. Nobody signs up to be a "worry wart," but having a healthy dose of concern and being proactive can be beneficial. Edward M. Hallowell, M.D., wrote a book entitled "Worry" and it explores every facet of this most common and debilitating emotional state. He contends that a healthy amount of concern can help us with job performance, anticipate potential dangers or threats, and learn from mistakes. In contrast, extreme forms of worry can become "toxic" and rob one of pleasurable experiences and self-sabotage our achievements. For example, if one is so worried about their academic performance, conducting a webinar, or winning a tennis match it can impact your performance in a negative manner.

The problem arises when one is unable to turn off worrisome thoughts. Some people experience anxiety attacks where they feel overwhelmed with panic and this can be frightening but can be effectively treated. Throughout my clinical experience, it appears that the majority of people who suffer from Generalized Anxiety Disorder or other forms of this diagnosis are incredibly intelligent and often times overachievers. Anxiety provoking situations that may occur in one's life such as divorce, relocating, or financial challenges can be managed better with physical activity. Mark Twain once said, "I've had a lot of worries in my life, most of which never happened." Toxic worry is counterproductive, but when you are exercising you may be able to assess if your ruminating thoughts are rational or simply toxic worry.

Exercise may give you a chance to restructure your cognitions and minimize toxic worry. The specific benefits are the changes in brain activity patterns that promote a sense of calm and well-being. Exercise releases endorphins, which are commonly referred to as the "feel good hormones" and are chemicals in your brain that energize your spirits and in general make you feel good. Finally, exercise allows you to put your mind in neutral mode and is part of one's self-care program.

Exercise Quotient (EQ): Chronic anxiety, worry, obsessive-compulsive tendencies, and panic attacks can improve with an exercise prescription.

Stress Busters: Exercise and Stress

Do you sometimes find it challenging to manage your personal and professional life? Due to stress you may feel overwhelmed, fatigued, have headaches, muscle cramps or your heart is racing? I like sending e-cards or cards to love ones and friends. I once saw a card that said, "I have to get out of these wet clothes and into a dry martini!" When you are stressed there may be a tendency to consume more alcohol or use it to take off the edge and sedate your stress. However, alcohol may not give you the desired effect you are seeking. Excessive drinking interferes with neurotransmitters in our brain that are needed for positive mental health. In some cases, alcohol consumption may impair good judgement, motor skills, poor impulse control, and lead to aggressive behavior.

In lieu of reaching for the cocktails to soothe your stress, go for a workout! Exercise is excellent for managing your stress. The physical activity promotes relaxation to the muscles and relieves the tension in the body. Stress is inevitable for all of us but incorporating aerobic activity has shown to improve your stress management. Your memory recall and cognitions function better since exercise stimulates the growth of new brain cells and helps prevent age-related decline. Self-esteem is boosted when one is exercising and you feel more confident and have improved self-efficacy. My clinical impressions are that people who exercise regularly feel they can manage their stress, acclimate to change, improve productivity, and have a satisfied sense of accomplishment.

Moreover, regular aerobic exercise will bring remarkable changes to your body, metabolism, heart, and your spirits. According to a Harvard study exercise has a unique capacity to exhilarate and relax, to provide stimulation and calm, and to dissipate stress. This study shows that the mental benefits of aerobic exercise have a neurochemical basis and exercise reduces levels of the body's stress hormones, such as adrenaline and cortisol. It stimulates the production of endorphins, chemicals in the brain that are the body's natural painkillers and mood elevators.

Working Up an Appetite: Exercise and Calories

A recent study shows that women spend an average of sixty-one minutes per day thinking about their food intake. Perhaps we focus on how many carbohydrates we consumed or have guilt about dining out for lunch and eating more than usual. Your mind starts racing with thoughts of how to conserve calories throughout the rest of the day or week. I've observed that these cognitions are even more prevalent for people who have formal eating disorders or are chronic dieters. Some people report that their thoughts about dieting, exercising, food intake, and body image consume them which leads to obsessionality.

The patients who stay in recovery and do not develop a second episode of an eating disorder and have better body image are the ones that seem to embrace exercise as a healthy habit. I believe the reasons for this are twofold: exercise improves psychological functioning (i.e., stress, depression and anxiety), and cognitive functioning (i.e., decrease in ruminating thoughts and obsessive-compulsive tendencies); and the physiological benefits (i.e., becoming more physically fit) are rewarding.

In my clinical experience, when one is exercising regularly one is not as consumed with thoughts about their caloric intake. It seems you can relax a bit and enjoy a dessert or not experience feelings of guilt or remorse after dining at a favorite restaurant. The positive body movement is helping others understand that we come in all shapes and sizes when it comes to body types.

Once you learn to implement intuitive eating you will be able to balance your food intake with your exercise regimen and minimize obsessive-compulsive thoughts. Furthermore, it seems easier and more manageable for most to stay in their healthy weight range when they are on an exercise program.

Foodies describe food in such a delectable style and truly enjoy the experience of gourmet dining. Food is viewed as an artistic pursuit that brings pleasure such as pairing a full-bodied cabernet with a Southwestern style steak. The bon appetite is part of this enlightened experience versus counting calories. Let's face it, many of us exercise so we can enjoy food and create an appetite. I am not referring to maladaptive behaviors and irrational thoughts such as "I will exercise to burn up my ingested calories." Every good meal or snack begins with hunger. The beauty of exercising is that once you establish your exercise regimen and know how many calories your body needs based on your metabolic rate, you will no longer count the calories, but learn to rely on cues for mindful eating.

Beautiful Body Satisfaction and Exercise

Many years ago, my niece told me that she has better body image when she is working out even if she sees only minimal changes in her body. She was on to something! Body dissatisfaction is often thought to be more prevalent for the female gender, but it does affect both genders. It has long been thought that body dissatisfaction is a precipitating factor for eating disorders and body dysmorphia. It seems that women and men in general are becoming increasingly dissatisfied with their body image. A new study conducted at the University of British Columbia examined the potential of physical activity to improve body image and the findings were published in the journal Psychology of Sport and Exercise. The physical self-perceptions and body images of women who exercised moderately for 30 minutes were compared with those who sat down to read.

The study assessed the "state body image," which is how one feels about one's body at a specific moment in time. The researchers examined the women's "physical self-efficacy," meaning how they felt about their general fitness, physical functioning, ability to perform tasks, physical self-perception, and affect. The women who worked out improved their body image significantly, compared to the ones that read and did not exercise. The effect was almost immediate and lasted for a minimum of 20 minutes after exercise. However, the affect and physical self-efficacy did not change significantly, but the self-perceptions of body fat and strength improved considerably post exercise. The positive effect did not seem to depend on mood changes but was due to the women seeing themselves as "stronger and thinner." The authors concluded the following: "We think that the feelings of strength and empowerment women achieve post exercise, stimulate an improved internal dialogue. This, in turn, should generate positive thoughts and feelings about their bodies which may replace the all too common negative ones."

EQ: Body dissatisfaction can be improved significantly through exercise as well as a more positive mental attitude.

Fit and Inspirational

Do you ever mimic a workout like one a celebrity does in hopes to have a body like them? Do you work out to lose weight or have a body like Kendal Jenner OR Jennifer Lopez? Many of us impose unrealistic expectations upon ourselves while exercising and it can lead to disappointment. A study revealed that fitspiration which can be defined as one focusing on an image with a message attached to that image may not be motivational. Actually, the study concluded that fitspiration messages should not be focused on during exercise. If you are imposing societal norms and expectations onto yourself during exercise it may be challenging to reap the other benefits of exercise.

Everyone seems to adore the talented actress Jennifer Lawrence because she is hilarious and relatable. When she won her first Oscar, she tripped prior to coming on stage and she seems to be able to roll with the punches! She will not succumb to the pressures of Hollywood and once stated, "I'm never going to starve myself for a part . . . I keep waiting for that one role to come along that scares me enough into dieting, and it just can't happen. I'm invincible." While she doesn't diet, Jennifer told Glamour, "I do exercise! You can't work when you're hungry, you know?" More impressively, she is an outstanding role model for young girls and women because she wants to set an example and she exudes strength and sincerity. Apparently when she trained for her role in Hunger Games, she never missed a workout and had a positive mental attitude which she seems to have in and out of the gym.

I challenge you to make a list of the benefits that will inspire you during your workout and to not include weight loss or emulating someone else's body. I am not suggesting that you may not experience more body satisfaction if you lose a few pounds or develop more muscle tone as an outcome of your exercise but shift the focus to health and wellness. Quite simply, the primary gain will be to improve physical and emotional well-being and secondary may be that you achieve your personal fitness goals and not others.

Timeless and Ageless: Exercise and Aging

Can you imagine answering the following questions without any emotional reaction: "How much do you weigh?" or "How old are you?" Yet we often learn other numerical facts about our health such as our blood pressure, heartrate, or body temperature without an emotional twinge. In some cultures, as one ages, they are respected more due to their acquired knowledge and wisdom. What if you began to see positive changes in your health and your annual physical exam after resuming an exercise program? If your blood pressure and heart rate are elevated and it drops significantly, this will serve as a positive reinforcement to maintain your exercise. In my opinion, if you want to look more youthful and radiant exercise can provide this for you. Moreover, you may no longer suffer from insomnia such as early morning awakenings or difficulty falling asleep. You are less fatigued and more energetic, and you have more time to devote to the activities that you love such as your family, friends, hobbies, or a charity.

One of the joys of being on campus at Cooper Aerobics Center is the attitude toward aging. The employees often say they are 40 years young versus 40 years old. Having a positive mental attitude about aging and seeing your health improve with exercise can be very inspiring. In fact, the Cooper Aerobics Institute now has established research on how long-term exercise improves your overall health and prevents many diseases. The Walker Wellness Clinic which is owned by my husband and myself, sets on this beautiful campus and the track runs throughout the campus with a lovely duck pond. Across the way you can see people playing a game of tennis or going for a swim. Throughout the day you may see members of the Cooper Fitness

Center going into the gym. Behind our clinic, is a school where children are playing on their playground and you can hear the sounds of their laughter.

I am amazed that we are surrounded by all ages. I watch members walk or run by on the track and I marvel at their compliance and level of fitness. As the years go by, I witness how one ages gracefully! Sometimes I see two women catching up on the latest news while walking together and enjoying the sunny day. There are men and women of all ages, but what inspires me the most are people 60 years of age and up exercising. I actually had the privilege of sitting next to a member that walks around the track daily at a fundraising dinner at the Cooper Institute and he was soon turning 100. He was charming, witty, and full of life! We had an interesting discussion and he actually had another engagement afterwards! Learning to embrace the aging process and viewing the cup as half full versus half empty, provides a positive mental attitude towards aging and exercising.

The Virgin Status:
Exercise and Physical Health Benefits

Many years ago, my husband and I underwent a comprehensive physical exam that was required for a new life insurance policy. After receiving my test results the insurance representative reported that I had a virgin status due to my positive test results. Afterwards, I reminded my husband quite often that he was married to a 47-year-old virgin! More importantly, for someone like myself who is not crazy about exercise, it inspired me to continue my exercise because it was working for me! One can find the physical benefits to be rewarding and motivational in spite of your feelings about exercise. If you are not at the point where you are committed to exercise, do it for your loved ones and eventually you will be doing it for yourself!

Similarly, the studies show that body esteem actually improves as one ages. Incorporating exercise into your lifestyle actually improves our body image and helps make one feel ageless. Some socially isolate if struggling with weight gain or the aging process, but exercise can help you not be as self-critical and self-deprecating about your body. As one ages typically your body esteem quotient (BEQ) improves and especially if you have worked on the quotients (i.e., psychological quotient, nutrition quotient, and exercise quotient)!

Exercise Quotient (EQ): Exercise improves body image as one ages and helps one embrace the aging process and not be so self-critical about their body.

Stretch like a Rubber band: Exercise and Stretching

Do you remember when you could easily do the splits if you were a cheerleader or dancer? Many of us do not take the time to incorporate stretching into our exercise routine. You want to get in and out of the gym and be done with your workout. The significance of stretching became more important for me after taking up piano lessons in my thirties. I realized that you can actually pull a muscle in one of your fingers if you do not warm up with scales and/or arpeggios. Stretching will eventually become second nature like brushing your teeth! Being flexible improves your movement at all ages and at all levels.

According to a study completed by Harvard University, stretching promotes flexibility and helps your joints maintain a healthy range of motion, and in doing so, also lowers the chances of joint and muscle strain. A panel of experts convened by the American College of Sports Medicine (ACSM) reviewed a wide range of studies to help answer these questions. Stretching has not been studied as much as other forms of exercise. However, based on the evidence, the panel agreed that healthy adults should do flexibility exercises (stretches or yoga) for all major muscle-tendon groups—neck, shoulders, chest, trunk, lower back, hips, legs, and ankles—at least two to three times a week. For optimal results, you should spend a total of sixty seconds on each stretching exercise. So, if you can hold a particular stretch for fifteen seconds, repeating it three more times would be ideal. If you can hold the stretch for twenty seconds, two more repetitions would do the trick.

The Balancing Act: Aerobic Conditioning and Strength Training Program

In order to improve your exercise quotient (EQ), you must find a balance between your strength training and aerobic conditions. According to the Cooper Institute studies, you should include endurance training such as walking, jogging, cycling, and swimming, plus muscle-building exercises. The muscle-building component might involve calisthenics, such as push-ups, sit-ups, pull-ups, or weight training of various types. The aerobic or cardio respiratory endurance component of your exercise is extremely important because of scientifically proven health and longevity benefits, which may not be associated with other types of exercise. The Cooper Institute studies have demonstrated that the more fit you are—as measured by treadmill stress-test times for fitness—the lower your risk will be for mortality from all causes. In other words, the higher your level of aerobic fitness, the less likely you are to die prematurely from a heart attack, cancer, diabetes, or any other cause.

As you age, the Cooper Institute recommends that the proportion of strength work should increase and by the time you turn sixty, your aerobic exercise should still constitute at least half of your routine. The purpose for this is that as you get older, your bone density naturally declines, and you are more at risk for osteoporosis, which strength training prevents by building up your bone mass. This danger of bone-thinning disease is especially serious for older women who are small-boned or have other risk factors, such as a fair complexion, northern European or Asian ethnic background, low percentage of body fat, and family history of bone disease. But the risk of a bone-loss disease is also very real for many men who are in their sixties or older. Completing bone density testing is crucial to monitor your bone health.

In addition, strength training helps you maintain tasks that may require the unusual muscle exertion like handling luggage. My husband and I visited Buenos Aires, Argentina, and Rio, Brazil and mastered the tango for our twentieth wedding anniversary. My objective was to have the endurance and stamina to do the cha cha, rhumba, and tango, all of which require good balance, strength, and flexibility. The fitter your muscles are, the lower your risk of pulling or straining a muscle, and you maintain better balance so you will avoid dangerous falls. All of our lessons and practice paid off, and it was a wonderful experience.

Exercise Prescription for Increasing Fitness by Philip Walker, MS, at Walker Wellness Clinic at Cooper Aerobics Center

I met my husband and business partner at Cooper Aerobics Center twenty-five years ago. He has had the privilege of designing exercise programs for patients in our clinic, professional golfers, athletes, and people who just want to become more physically fit. He once designed an exercise prescription for the oldest man to climb Mount Everest. The beauty of the exercise prescription he designed below is that it can be adaptable to any environment or situation.

Exercise Prescription for Optimal Fitness

Go Faster, Go Longer, Have More Strength, and Touch Your Toes!

Frequency: 3 to 5 days per week
Duration: 15 to 60 minutes per session for 3–4 days, 20–90 minutes for one day
Type: Maximum
- 5 Aerobic training sessions
- 2 Stretching sessions.
- 2 Strength training sessions,

Aerobic training: Whatever you find enjoyable and convenient such as:
- Walking (self, friend, or treadmill), jogging (outdoors, indoors, pool), swimming, rope jumping, stair stepping/climbing, cycling (outside, home, gym, spinning), rowing (home, lake, gym), roller blading, dancing, Jumping jacks, Elliptical, water aerobics, gardening, boxing.

Strength Training:
- Outside—Benches, picnic tables, bands, trees, sticks, rocks, grass, bricks, walls, bars (not drinking type), hills, and banks
- Indoors—free weights (recommended), bands, chairs, tables, floor, fire logs, cans of food, books, sand bags, stairs, spouse!
- Gym/Fitness Center—personal trainer, free weights, machine weights.
- Flexibility Exercises:
- Yoga mat, carpet, grass, park, table, bench, wall, tree, chair, door, patio, bed

Day 1: (total time: 25–45minutes)
- A. Warm-up: 3–5 minutes (slow to light pace pre-aerobic exercise)
- B. Aerobic phase: (activity of choice) 15–30 minutes; gradually increasing speed over set distance or number by 5 to 15 seconds each week
- C. Cool down: 2–3 minutes (slow to light pace)
- D. Strength training: 5–10 minutes—Start at comfortable weight/repetitions/angle for each exercise. Your goal is to increase either/or weight/repetitions/angle every two weeks.
- E. Stretching Exercises: 2–5 minutes

Exercise Prescription for Optimal Fitness (cont.)

Day 2: (total time: 30–40 minutes)
  A. Warm-up: 3–5 minutes (slow to light pace pre-aerobic activity)
  B. Aerobic Phase: (activity of choice) 20–30 minutes at comfortable/brisk pace
  C. Cool down: 2–3 minutes (slow to light pace)
  D. Stretching Exercises: 5–10 minutes

Day 3: (total time: 25–45minutes)
  A. Warm-up: 3–5 minutes (slow to light pace pre-aerobic activity)
  B. Aerobic Phase: 20 to 30 minutes fartlek (speed play) training. Increase speed (to fast pace) varying between 20–60 seconds per sprint to increase heart rate. Return to a comfortable pace before repeating. Complete 5 to 8 sprints
  C. Strength: 5–10 minutes Start at comfortable weight/repetitions/angle for each exercise. Your goal is to increase either/or weight/repetitions/angle every two weeks.
  D. Stretching Exercises: 2–5 minutes

Day 4: (total time: 30–45 minutes)
  A. Warm-up: 3–5 minutes (slow to light pace pre-aerobic activity)
  B. Aerobic Phase: (activity of choice) 20–30 minutes at comfortable/brisk pace
  C. Cool down: 2–3 minutes (slow to light pace)
  D. Stretching Exercises: 5–10 minutes

Day 5: (total time 20–95 minutes)
  A. Aerobic Phase: Activity(s) of choice at comfortable pace commencing 20—30 minutes. Increase activity(s) each week by 3–5 minutes until you can comfortably achieve continuous activity(s) for 90 minutes.
  B. Stretching Exercises: 3- 5 minutes

Notes: If you have limited days to exercise, the following is recommended:
  • 1 day/week complete—complete Day 3
  • 2 days/week complete—complete Days 3 and 5
  • 3 days/week complete—complete Days 1, 3, and 5
  • 4 days/week complete—complete Days 1, 2, 3 and 5

Uniquely You: Exercise for Yourself

Exercise becomes more meaningful if you eventually come to the conclusion that you are doing it for yourself! However, if you are able to see the positive results in your mental and physical health, you may have a greater appreciation for physical activity. Positive reinforcements may keep you engaged like rewarding yourself with a manicure and pedicure or downloading new iTunes or eBooks. I often notice that Starbuck's is packed mid-morning, and many of the customers are dressed in workout clothes! Treat yourself or join a friend afterwards at your favorite coffee shop, and enjoy your signature flavor! Our patients seem more committed to exercise if they actually put it in their smart phone or calendar and exercise for self-care.

In summary, one of the most significant reasons for improving your exercise quotient is to realize that you are uniquely different than others, and you may require more or less exercise depending on biological and genetic factors. Therefore, it is important to maintain your healthy body weight range, caloric intake, and exercise prescription to improve your metabolism and body esteem. The task may be somewhat daunting at first, but it will eventually become second nature when you fall into a comfortable plan that works for your body type. You will find your rhythm as your implement mindful eating (NQ) with your exercise prescription (EQ) since the two go hand and hand and complement one another.

Chapter 5
Nutrition: Piece of Cake

*"Strength is the capacity to break a chocolate
bar in four pieces and eat just one."*
—Judith Viorst

*I*t is your birthday, and you want to celebrate in style! Did you know
that there is an annual international cake competition where clever
cake design is celebrated? Birthday cakes are often enjoyed not only for
the festive decoration, but also because they mark your special day! And
most of us want to be able to enjoy a piece of our favorite birthday cake
such as that delicious traditional birthday cake from your favorite bakery
with a scoop of ice cream. *It feels like such a treat!* Now, think about times
when you've celebrated birthdays. Did you experience any guilt before,
during, or after having a piece of that delicious cake, or did you have your
piece of cake and also enjoy peace of mind?

More recently, emotions such as guilt, which can be a symptom of
depression, are associated with food than ever before. We have established
that we often approach our food intake in a dichotomous manner: whether
we label it as a "bad food" or a "good food" (i.e., "I was really bad because
I ate pasta and mostly carbs."). But, many of us today have picked up labels
for food based on trends, diets, and conversations that we have had with

others about what you "should" and "shouldn't" be eating. By not attaching derogatory labels to yourself and your food, you will improve your body esteem. My approach to eating is focused on balanced nutrition. When the goal is to balance the food you eat in order to provide nourishment for your body, you will discover that you can have your cake and eat it too. In this chapter, we will focus on remaking your experience with food and offer up a sense of freedom to make eating a pleasurable experience.

There is much to be learned from studying the relationship of shame and guilt in eating behaviors. The words *shame* and *guilt* are often used interchangeably; however, from a psychological perspective, it is important to make the distinction between the terms. Guilt represents how we feel about ourselves, whereas shame is being cognizant of the fact one may have injured another person. According to *Psychology Today* guilt is a feeling of responsibility or remorse for some offense whether it be real or imagined. Shame is defined as the painful feeling arising from the awareness of something dishonorable done by oneself or another. In the case of fat shaming or body shaming, I think it is a cruel and unkind act. As a clinician, I encourage my patients to be accountable for their behavior but not impose guilt or shame upon themselves or others.

In a study with Australian women exhibiting eating disorder symptoms, the objective was to predict the severity of eating disturbance and the proneness to shame and guilt associated specifically with eating contexts, and shame associated with the body. The study also sought to determine if shame is a more prominent emotion than guilt among women who have eating difficulties. The results showed that shame associated with eating behavior was the strongest predictor of the severity of eating disorder symptoms. Other predictors were guilt associated with eating behavior and body shame.

How do we make peace with that "piece of cake"? Some may interpret this as it is best to avoid all foods that create shame and guilt, but this chapter will help you eat in a responsible and healthy way without inducing guilt and shame while allowing you to enjoy more indulgent foods when you choose to have them. The key word here is "choice." Many of us too often feel that making decisions about what to eat as more of a burden than a choice. Food is not the enemy! It is simply a choice and one that is a crucial part of living, so the sooner we make peace with it, the sooner you can just eat your birthday cake and freely celebrate with friends and family on your birthday!

The Four F's: Food, Feelings, Fuel, and Frequency

Food and Feelings

As you focus on your food intake and nutrition, it is important to identify the four F's: Food, Feelings, Fuel, and Frequency. As we have established, if you are experiencing stress, you may crave carbohydrates which actually soothe our stress level. According to a study published in July 2000 *American Demographics*, "People in happy moods tended to prefer foods such as pizza or steak (32%), sad people reached for ice cream and cookies (39%), and bored people opened up a bag of potato chips (36%)." This study proposed that salty equals boredom; crunchy equals anger or frustration; spicy equals excitement or intensity; sweet equals joy and contentment.

NQ: Learn to identify specific feelings that may lead to emotional eating by using the hunger rating scale and becoming psychologically introspective.

Food and Fuel

The purpose of food is to provide nourishment and fuel to our bodies. Imagine that your body is a finely tuned automobile; it is important to keep the engine running, do maintenance, and keep it clean. You would not want your car to run out of gas and leave you stranded on the side of the road, so now we have friendly reminders like those warning lights, to tell us when your fuel is getting low. Your body needs to be treated with at least the same care that you provide for your beloved car, which simply means that it is important to provide proper nutrition and stay well hydrated. Unlike your car, which you will eventually trade in for a newer model, your body is your vehicle for life. Proper fuel keeps the engine running smoothly. Our goal here is to be able to identify the times that you need nourishment and how to use food choice to take care of your life machine: your body.

NQ: Fuel your body for nourishment and energy expended and adjust to your needs as you would fuel a beloved and valuable luxury vehicle.

Food and Frequency

Frequent feedings are the best way to manage your weight and stay in a healthy weight range. Starving your body or restricting your food intake actually slows down the metabolism and sets you up for a weight gain. It is typically recommended to eat every three to five hours. Researchers have known for years that fullness after a meal is only one aspect of feeling satisfied. Studies suggest that leptin also interacts with the neurotransmitter dopamine in the brain to produce a feeling of pleasure after eating. The brain must receive a signal from the digestive hormones secreted by the gastrointestinal tract. Your brain and stomach register feelings of fullness after about twenty minutes. Slow down the eating process by setting down your utensils, chewing slowly, savoring your meal, sipping your beverage, and enjoying dinner conversation.

During this time, receptors inform the brain that your body is receiving nutrients by sending hormone signals. The hormone cholecystokinin is released by your intestines, and the hormone leptin tells your brain about your long-term needs and overall satiety based on how much energy your body is storing. Visualize this as having a live chat online. Leptin may amplify the signals that cholecystokinin sends to enhance your sense of fullness, and it may help the neurotransmitter dopamine give you feelings of pleasure after eating. As with all effective communication, one needs to learn to be an active listener, be patient, and avoid interrupting the other party. If you eat too fast, these hormones may not have enough time to properly communicate.

The theory is that by eating too quickly, people may not give this intricate hormonal cross-talk system enough time to work. It is analogous to sending a text message and not waiting for the response. Some may suffer from what is known as leptin resistance, which means that one may not be reaching satiety or receive the signals from the hormones described above. Yet taking more time to complete these signals can be a learned process and skill that one can acquire over time.

NQ: Practice implementing the hormonal cross talk described above and over time you will establish habitual eating patterns, so you not only reach satiety, but the feelings of enjoying your food.

Queen Bee

Although I respect the Queen of England, I find it fascinating that while dining, the royal family looks to the queen to begin eating each course, and all are required to mimic her eating style. This potentially means that the royal family may be consuming the same amount of caloric intake as the queen. At ninety-two, the queen still rides horses, but her metabolism has probably slowed down with age, and she may not be participating in a vigorous exercise regimen like many of those who dine with her who more than likely need more calories than the Queen. Everyone's caloric needs differ according to their metabolism, exercise intake, and other variables. Therefore, it is unrealistic to use another person as your model for eating.

In fact, one key element to remember is that you, and only you, are responsible for your nutrition intake and the choices and speed at which you consume your food. Allowing others to control or reprimand your choices and style of eating sets up a power and control dynamic in the relationship that is counterproductive. I give you permission to fire your food police and take personal responsibility for yourself when it comes to managing your nutrition. One may have a tendency to overeat after dieting due to deprivation or restriction. In addition, it is important that you learn to not overestimate or underestimate your food intake. Perhaps visualizing your food groups on your plate will help you be cognizant of serving sizes in lieu of the laborious task of counting every morsel you put in your mouth. These techniques allow you to normalize your eating and become more confident in the fact that you've got this, and you are personally accountable for the choices you make. That encourages a much more powerful and productive feeling than questioning or shaming every bite you eat.

NQ: Pace your eating to allow your mind to receive a message approximately twenty minutes after you begin eating that you are full, and fire the food police.

A Calorie Is a Calorie Is a Calorie

Many of us are very confused when it comes to nutrition as the trends seem to change as quickly as fashion designs. Most of us have googled the calorie count of various foods, but according to Huffpost, google recently announced America's ten top trending calorie count searches of 2016, and the results were somewhat surprising. The findings were astonishing since only one in five millennials have tried a Big Mac, but this was on the list. Quinoa, which has made the list, is considered a supergrain and has increased in popularity more recently because it is high in dietary fiber. Dietitians recommend consuming at least 25 grams of fiber per day and quinoa contains 5 grams of fiber, which makes it a great choice for a source of fiber.

Another one that made the list was white wine, which is an average of 121 calories per glass. Conversely, red wine is approximately 126 calories per glass. Interestingly enough, some people do not factor in alcoholic calories, but they should be considered because they do count. The idea of counting your alcohol calories may help one moderate their alcohol intake. It is important to be aware that one can become cross addicted (i.e., switching from food addiction to alcohol addiction).

At the end of the day "a calorie is a calorie is a calorie." A calorie may be defined as a unit of energy. In nutrition and everyday language, calories refer to energy consumption through eating and drinking, and energy usage through physical activity. For example, an apple may have 80 calories, while a 1-mile walk might use up about 100 calories.

All of us require different amounts of calories to maintain, gain, or lose weight, and no resting metabolic rate is the same. Your resting metabolic rate is the number of calories you burn a day to maintain body function. Caloric intake may vary due to genetic predispositions, biological factors, medical diagnoses, and history of dieting among other variables. Counting calories can be a slippery slope if you have obsessive-compulsive tendencies, but being cognizant of the number of calories you consume every day is essential.

Consuming too few calories may slow down your metabolism and make you vulnerable for a future weight gain. On the other hand, ingesting a higher level of calories than your body may need could create a weight gain. If you observe babies and toddlers, you will notice that, for the most part, they are mindful eaters because they eat when they are hungry and stop when they are full. My philosophy is that disordered eating comes from the food rules that we allow society to impose upon us and that we eventually impose on ourselves. Restore the joy of eating while training yourself to be mindful of your caloric intake, and you can loosen the grip that collected food rules gathered along the way may have had on you. Here are a few that you may have collected that you now need to just let go:

Food Rules

- Thou shall not eat in between meals.
- Desserts are forbidden.
- Good girls do not eat chocolate.
- Thou should eat the same amount as others.
- If you drink alcohol for your dinner you should not eat.
- You must avoid dairy products.
- Don't eat now; it will spoil your dinner.
- How can you be hungry; you just ate!
- Clean your plate!
- Kids are starving so don't waste your food.
- If you start eating, you may not be able to stop.
- I must weigh myself every day to determine what I can eat.
- Carbohydrates make you fat.
- Omit fat from your diet.

The Foodie

Do you ever marvel at the way a chef or foodie describe their food? If you watch the Food Network, you hear chefs like Giada de Laurentis and Bobby Flay characterize their food with adjectives such as "it has great texture" or "a wonderful depth of flavor." What about other descriptions such as "a party in my mouth" or "the warmth from cinnamon and nutmeg." There is a certain amount of pride and respect that is shown toward food when one is a foodie. Along the way many of us have learned to speak about food in a derogatory fashion: "Adding nuts gives it a great crunch factor, but they are too fattening." I am suggesting that we begin to talk about food with excitement and not disdain.

The communication style in categorizing our food with dichotomous thinking such as "fattening or healthy" seems to have a significant impact on cognitive functioning (e.g., pizza is bad for me because it makes me fat.) One begins to label themselves as well as their food with negative connotations. If you have labeled all fats as unhealthy or carbohydrates as causing weight gain, you probably have more mental preoccupation with these food groups. When you speak negatively about your food, it has a negative correlation with your body image. Learn to speak respectfully about yourself and your food, and you will not only have a positive attitude toward yourself, but toward the foods you consume. Show your food some RESPECT, and you will receive more self-respect. The following are examples of how to help you talk about food and take a moment to substitute the ingredients or recipes in your own words. Change your "food rules" to "food talk."

Food Talk

- The cilantro in the guacamole on my toast is delicious and sustains me until lunch time.
- Tomato basil soup and grilled cheese with gruyere are a perfect pair, especially on a cold winter's night when I am craving something warm.
- Country cooking like black eyed peas, okra, squash, and potatoes reminds me of the garden we had growing up and my mother's wonderful cooking.
- Afternoon tea with ginger biscuits and tea sandwiches is such a lovely British tradition.
- My favorite dinner is fresh lobster with lemon butter because it is reminiscent of spending time with friends in Maine and viewing the picturesque fall foliage.

Food preferences are foods that you prefer over others and sometimes it is important to choose your foods wisely based on the ones you really like. If you avoid all food cravings at all times, you may not feel satisfied and actually consume more calories. Perhaps you are tempted to eat around your cravings versus satisfying them. If you are craving an oatmeal and raisin cookie and you eat raisins instead followed a bowl of oatmeal with maple syrup and butter, and then other foods, it would be so much easier to have that cookie you were craving since you will experience satisfaction. Below are some examples of food preferences, and I challenge you to substitute the language based on your favorite foods.

Food Preferences:

- I prefer Thai food over Indian food.
- I prefer a dessert that has chocolate in lieu of fruit.
- I prefer light and creamy peanut butter over regular crunchy peanut butter.

Food Dislikes:

- I do not enjoy eating pickled beets, but I love them roasted.
- I do not like vanilla ice cream by itself, but I like it on cobblers or crisp.
- I do not like fast food, but I love sliders on the grill.

Creating Memories and Traditions

Many memories, holidays, and traditions allow us to celebrate with food. Memories are to be cherished and can be an opportunity to spice up your life! Allow yourself to recall the aromas of your kitchen when you were a child and connect with some memories that you want to savor as an adult. These memories bring us comfort and happiness. Or you may want to create new memories around new foods. You may recall the aroma of your mother's roasted chicken and vegetables that permeated the kitchen or the spices of a homemade apple pie. Below is a list of food memories and traditions that my husband and I celebrate annually. I challenge you to substitute words that describe your own memories from the past and make new ones for the future. In fact, if you state the memory you want to create, it will help you envision the experience, and you can fuel the desire and the specifics to actualize what you envision.

Our anniversary is celebrated by visiting a new country like Switzerland where we can enjoy the food and culture.

Thanksgiving dinner is Southwestern stuffing, Cornish hens, cranberry mold, and chocolate chip cheesecake.

Valentine's Day is filled with roses, champagne, and a dark orange chocolate fountain for dipping strawberries!

I bake luscious lemon tea cakes in the shape of hearts and roses and serve them with tea when our British family visits us!

What's for Dinner?

We've all had those moments when you try to decide what you want for dinner. There are so many options today, whether it be dining out or sipping a glass of wine as you prepare a lovely meal. Many factors go into our decision making regarding dinner plans or meal planning in general. There are methods to help you incorporate your food groups into meal planning whether you are eating on the run as you catch your next flight or preparing meals for a family that has different schedules due to work and extracurricular activities.

Moreover, having a well-stocked pantry, refrigerator, and freezer filled with favorites allows you to have a wonderful and stress-free dining experience. It is not advisable to allow yourself to run out of food choices. Many dieters limit what they bring into their kitchen to have better impulse control, but I am suggesting just the opposite. Gradually introduce foods that you perceive as forbidden so over time you learn to trust yourself and gain control by not overeating or feeling deprived. However, the objective is to stock your kitchen with the foods you love and learn to gradually improve your ability to moderate your food intake! After all, the process of eating produces the endorphin effect and should be an enjoyable event. Therefore, it is essential to select foods that tingle your taste buds and please your palate when you are preparing your dinner or meals in general.

My experience of waiting tables in college opened my eyes to how many people become irritable before dinnertime. I learned very quickly that if there was a crying baby to get some crackers and the bread basket to the table immediately. If you allow your blood sugar levels to get too low and you become ravenous, you are not honoring your hunger sensation. You are teaching your body and brain to distrust that you know when to eat. In planning ahead, it is important to feed yourself every three to five hours to regulate your blood sugar level and stabilize your mood. If your meal contained minimal fat or protein, you may experience a hunger sensation more quickly and can allow yourself to have a snack prior to the next meal. If you have had a meal with higher fat and protein, intake you may be comfortably full for longer. Keep food with you at all times to avoid these moments where your blood sugar drops and you feel light headed because this feeling often leads to overeating.

Frequent feedings where you have access to a snack such as nuts, fruits, or cheese allows you to steadily feel satisfied. Once you normalize your eating, you may find you have food left over when you complete a meal. Now don't let that activate guilt about wasting food! Over time, as you retrain yourself, you'll have balance in all areas that touch your food experience. If you have planned a sandwich, soup, fruit, and milk for lunch and you are comfortably full before you finish your fruit, save it for your afternoon snack. Tune in to your feelings of hunger and satiety. It may feel like a roller coaster at first, but soon your body will get the message that it can eat when hungry.

In addition, consuming your food in a pleasant environment such as a park or away from technology, sets the mood for you to be an intuitive eater and not disassociate while you are eating. Take a moment to reflect on all of the places where you can have your dinner: your favorite seafood restaurant, kitchen nook on taco night, formal dining room table with a candle-lit dinner with spaghetti and meatballs, throw some kabobs on the grill and eat outdoors, a panini party at your bar, or a cozy fireside dinner with homemade butternut squash soup. Consuming your food in a tranquil environment allows you to be in touch with the "hear and now" and experience a food-induced state of euphoria. Enjoy it!

NQ: Learn to regulate your blood sugar levels and mood by eating every three to five hours and implementing frequent feeding to stabilize your blood sugar and stay in your healthy weight range.

Nutrition Quotient Questionnaire

Take a moment to complete the nutrition quotient questionnaire below to increase your knowledge on nutrition

1. In general, the correlation between food and emotions is

   _____ Not significant

   _____ Very significant

   _____ Has not been researched

   _____ Is a joke

2. In the past thirty years the percent of fat in the American diet has:

   _____ Increased

   _____ Decreased

   _____ Has had no increase or decrease

   _____ Has reached an all-time high

3. If you are the same age and gender as another person you will need

   _____ More calories

   _____ Exact amount of exercise

   _____ Less calories

   _____ Different amounts of calories based on your metabolism

4. Eating frequently is a good way to

   _____ Maintain your weight

   _____ Gain weight

   _____ Stabilize blood sugar levels and mood

   _____ Become obese

5. The food pyramid contains the following food groups except

   _____ Peanut butter and jelly

   _____ Protein

   _____ Dairy

   _____ Carbohydrates

6. Fear foods are

_____ Good for your health

_____ Ones you fear and avoid due to concerns about weight gain

_____ Eaten on Halloween

_____ Consumed in the presence of others

7. Carbohydrates are

_____ The body's main source of energy

_____ Should be avoided at all cost

_____ Most of the calories needed

_____ Only recommended for children

8. Protein is a structural component of muscle tissues, organs and cell walls and

_____ Is a backup source of energy once carbohydrates and fat are no longer available

_____ Should be 15 to 20 percent of your calories consumed

_____ It can be found in fish, chicken, beans, and tofu

_____ All of the above

9. Calories eaten in the evening are

_____ More fattening than calories eaten in the day time

_____ The reason for weight gain

_____ No more fattening and what matters is your overall caloric intake

_____ The ones you should focus on exclusively for your nutrition intake

10. Chronic dieting

_____ Leads to weight gain over time

_____ Slows down your metabolism

_____ Is the reason that most people (about 95%) regain their weight

_____ All of the above

11. Omitting food groups

_____ Such as carbohydrates is necessary

_____ Is recommended by the American Dietetic Association

_____ Is unhealthy because your body needs the vitamins and minerals from all food groups

_____ Helps you lose weight

12. Consuming fat does all of the following for our bodies except

_____ Should be no more than 10 percent of your calories

_____ Maintains hair, nail and skin health

_____ Provides protection from injury (i.e., internal organs, bones)

_____ Provides proper cellular function

13. Eating most of your calories

_____ In the daytime helps you maintain your weight

_____ In the evening creates a weight gain

_____ Before 6:00 P.M. and not afterwards is advisable

_____ Throughout the day and evening does not create a weight gain

14. Carbohydrates and sugars create

_____ A weight gain

Do not cause weight gain unless they contribute to excess calorie intake

_____ An unhealthy relationship with food

Are the only way to sustain weight loss long term

You can find the answers at www.bodyesteem.com

Food Groups

Carbohydrates Are Not the Enemy

The question arises whether carbohydrates are our friends or foe. Carbohydrates are actually our friend and not our enemy. Many people fear carbohydrates and having tried various low-carb diets, periodically restrict their carbohydrate consumption. But even when they aren't restricting carbs, they often feel guilty about eating them. Allowing yourself to enjoy a treat (a simple carbohydrate) is perfectly acceptable within moderation. Our licensed registered dieticians often recommend adding a simple carbohydrate (e.g., two chocolate chip cookies) into patient's daily routine to satisfy cravings. It works beautifully so the patient does not experience deprivation, which is a prelude to overeating. Carbohydrates are one of the primary types of nutrients and the one needed in the largest amounts by the body. Carbohydrates are often considered a contributing factor for weight gain, but your body needs carbohydrates to fuel physical activity as well as brain and organ function. Therefore, it is important to never omit carbs as a food group from your nutrition plan. Instead, choose them wisely and for the nutritional value they offer.

NQ: Carbohydrates are necessary to provide energy and as a source of fuel that you need for physical activity and healthy brain and organ function and should never be omitted or overly restricted from your nutrition plan.

You may have heard that simple carbohydrates are synonymous with simple sugars (which are very low in nutritional value) and are typically found in high concentrations in foods and beverages such as sodas that contain sugar or sports drinks, candy, and pastries. Unlike complex carbohydrates there are not as many vitamins, minerals, phytochemicals (non-nutrients in plant-based foods that help prevent disease) or much fiber.

Perhaps this is a valid reason to choose your carbohydrates wisely, but do not become too restrictive if you enjoy the aforementioned simple carbohydrates. Complex carbohydrates are plant-based foods, and include things such as fruits and vegetables, and whole grains. Moreover, with the exception of fruit, legumes such lentils and beans are a great source of protein as well.

Carbohydrates are not your nemesis. Since carbohydrates are the main fuel for exercise, consuming your carbohydrates as complex carbs is a great eating strategy because not only do carbohydrates fuel your exercise, afterward your muscles can store carbohydrates and protein as energy and help in recovery.

You can gain weight from eating excessive amounts of carbohydrates, but it is important to remember that your body weight status is dictated by the number of calories you consume each day versus the number of calories you expend. If you enjoy simple carbohydrates, allow yourself a designated amount (a scoop of cookie dough ice cream) in your daily dietary intake.

In essence, approach your food intake like your bank account in a responsible manner analogous to being fiscally competent. You certainly wouldn't want to charge your credit card with an amount you cannot afford to pay off at the end of the month. Any excess results in paying interest, which begins to drag on your finances over time. Consuming excessive amounts of calories, even the ones that you deem healthy, can result in weight gain if you consume more calories than needed to fuel your energy expenditure. Being mindful of the quality of the calories and carbohydrates you are consuming also adds quality to your fuel. In general, the Cooper Institute reports that by limiting simple carbohydrates and emphasizing complex carbohydrates in our diet, we significantly decrease our risk for developing type 2 diabetes, as well as cardiovascular disease, diverticulitis, and some cancers. Furthermore, these risks can be decreased further by becoming more physically active and maintaining a healthy body weight range. I hope you will enjoy recipes from my upcoming cookbook. The one below is one of our favorite carbohydrates that is a Thanksgiving tradition.

Southwestern Stuffing

My husband and I made this on our first Thanksgiving together, and we enjoy it throughout the winter. We now reflect and laugh at how inexperienced we were as cooks. Serves approximately 15 cups.

Corn bread mix

1 cup of corn kernels (roasted)
6 tablespoons of unsalted butter
1 ½ cups of chopped red onions
1 ½ cup of assorted colors of chopped bell peppers
4 large poblano chilies (seeded and chopped)
2 pickled jalapeno chilies (finely chopped)
¼ cup of chopped fresh sage
1 ½ cup of fresh oregano
1 bunch of cilantro
1 ½ cup of crushed Frito-Lays
1 ¼ cup of cream style corn
3 large eggs beaten or egg beaters

Bake cornbread per instructions. Preheat oven to 500 degrees and roast the corn kernels (not the cream style corn) with cooking spray and cayenne pepper and stir occasionally. Allow the corn to cool and then adjust the oven to 350 degrees to cook the stuffing.

Chop the vegetables in a fine size using an alligator chopper or another vegetable chopper to save time. Over medium heat sauté all vegetables and herbs except for the cilantro in a skillet for approximately 15–20 minutes or until tender. Allow to cool before adding to the cornbread. Mix in cilantro, corn chips, corn kernels, cream style corn, and eggs. If the mixture is too dry, add more cream style corn. If it is too moist, add more corn chips. Season with salt and pepper. Mix well. Bake stuffing inside Cornish hens, turkey, or in a buttered baking dish. Coat foil with cooking spray, cover and bake 40 minutes. Uncover and bake until the top begins to brown, about 15 minutes.

The Dairy King and Queen

After traveling to England, the last twenty-five years to visit my in laws I have learned a great deal about English traditions such as afternoon tea, opening crackers that contain paper crowns, and riddles on Christmas Day and Boxing Day (the day after Christmas when the staff receive their gifts). However, did you know that the royals are not permitted to be photographed while they are eating? Why would such a normal activity as consuming your food not be photographed?

In America, we don't have a royal family, but I challenge you to become a dairy king and queen by making sure that you get your three servings of dairy on a daily basis. Many people started to eliminate or reduce the amount of dairy in their diet as result of following a low-fat plan. Again, balanced eating is the best approach and strictly limiting any food group results in nutritional deficits.

Today, most of us receive very little sun exposure due to the risk factors associated with cancer. Being a sun goddess is no longer healthy, but it has become somewhat challenging to get the benefits of vitamin D, which is commonly referred to as the sunshine vitamin and is produced by the body in response to skin being exposed to sunlight.

A Web M.D. study reported that if you have milk allergies, adhere to a strict vegan diet, and lack of sun exposure, you may be at risk for vitamin

D deficiency. The study also revealed that vitamin D occurs naturally in some foods such as fish, fish liver oils, egg yolks, and in fortified dairy and grain products. In addition, vitamin D is essential for strong bones, because it helps the body use calcium from the diet. Increasingly research is revealing the importance of vitamin D in protecting against health complications (i.e., bone pain and muscle weakness, increased risk of death and cardiovascular problems, cognitive impairment in older adults, asthma in children, and cancer). The benefits of bone health are simply amazing! It is imperative to incorporate dairy into your dietary intake since this study reported that ten million Americans suffer from osteoporosis and an additional forty-three million are at risk of developing the condition.

Women are four times more likely to develop osteoporosis, but older men are also susceptible. Although more research is needed to understand the role of dietary protein on bone health, studies show the protein and calcium in milk may play a critical role in bone health and density, thereby decreasing the risk for osteoporosis. Three daily servings of low-fat or fat-free dairy provide essential nutrients that work together to build strong bones.

Furthermore, foods that contain dairy products are an essential source of nutrients for all ages and especially for children and adolescents. If you suffer from lactose intolerance, this means that you have an insufficient level of the lactase enzyme that breaks down lactose, which is the naturally occurring sugar found in most dairy foods. There are other options for you to get your calcium via lactose-free milk. You will enjoy your milk again without the symptoms with digestion that cause discomfort from being lactose intolerant.

NQ: Incorporate vitamin D into your nutritional intake since most of us are deficient in this vitamin, and it protects and prevents health complications such as osteoporosis or osteopenia, cognitive impairment in older adults, risk for death and cardiovascular disease, asthma in children, and cancer.

If you do not like milk, there are myriad ways you can consume your daily requirement without consuming milk. Next time you toss your salad, sprinkle on a serving of goat cheese or feta. One of my favorite ways to entertain is to set up appetizers where you can assemble your own which gives the guests a chance to chat as they make their choices. In Texas we often say "Belly up to the bar," but this is not a cocktail bar; it is bar food. Other great appetizers are creating a satay bar with shrimp, beef, or chicken and serving my homemade peanut sauce and other Asian sauces. It is easy to eat because it is skewered, and all you need is a cocktail napkin. A Swiss fondue on a lazy Susan with crudité for dipping is another fun culinary experience as well as a deviled egg bar with toppings such as crab, chives, or smoked salmon. At any rate, it seems our family's and friends' favorite is a bruschetta bar, and it happens to be mine as well!

Sun-Dried Tomato and Basil Bruschetta

In Italy, most restaurants serve bruschetta, and during our travels we sampled this delectable appetizer. Use your imagination to come up with a variety of toppings! Serves approximately 24.

8.5-ounce jar of sun-dried tomatoes in olive oil
24 thin slices of a whole grain French baguette
½ cup of fresh basil
8 ounces of goat cheese
Other varieties: basil pesto with a sprinkle of parmesan cheese; stilton cheese with pear and walnuts

Drain the olive oil from the sun-dried tomatoes and reserve the oil. Cut the sun-dried tomatoes in small pieces. Use a pastry brush to brush the baguette slices with the sun-dried tomato olive oil. Toast at 425 degrees for just a few minutes on each side of the bread. Spread goat cheese on the baguette slices, and top with the sun-dried tomatoes. Place in the oven again with the same temperature for approximately 2–5 minutes and monitor carefully. Chiffonade the basil and place on top of the bruschetta and serve.

Protein: Moo Moo, Quack Quack, Something Fishy, Veggilicious, Veganize Me

As kids we often played the game where you made sounds of different animals such as the cow says, "moo moo" and the duck says, "quack quack," and so on. We didn't realize that we were actually learning about various types of protein that we may consume. Protein is a macronutrient and food group that is vital for nutrition intake, and it certainly keeps our tummy full. There are so many options today that it is challenging to know what type of protein that one can consume since "eggs are an eggcellent choice," vegetarians and vegans consume beans and tofu, and plenty of Texans go for a juicy red steak as enthusiastic carnivores.

Who am I to recommend the method by which you choose your protein? You may choose from being a pescatarian, vegetarian, carnivore, or vegan. In our clinics we honor patients' choices as long as they are getting the nutrients and vitamins they need according to their nutritional analysis. If a patient is vegan or vegetarian, we have them complete a nutritional analysis to assess the appropriate amount of protein their bodies need as well as other vitamins and minerals. Perhaps a quick education on the benefits of protein may help you make your choices for the best quality of protein.

Protein is found in muscle, bone, skin, hair, and virtually every other body part or tissue. At least 10,000 different proteins make you what you are and keep you that way. However, millions of people are getting inadequate amounts of protein in their daily diet. Lack of protein can cause growth failure, loss of muscle mass, decreased immunity, weakening of the heart and respiratory system, and even death. So, it is vital that you incorporate protein into your daily dietary intake.

Seafood

Do you remember the seafood diet: I see food and I eat it? We now know that seafood is an excellent source of protein because it's usually low in fat. Fish such as salmon is a little higher in fat, but it is heart healthy and has omega-3 fatty acids.

White Meat Poultry

White meat poultry is a great choice since it is considered lean protein. Dark meat is a little higher in fat, but you may prefer the taste over white meat. You may or may not want to remove the skin since it is loaded with saturated fat.

Milk, Cheese, and Yogurt

Dairy foods like milk, cheese, and yogurt are sources of protein, contain calcium, and many are fortified with vitamin D. Choose skim or low-fat dairy products as a prevention of osteopenia and osteoporosis and for strong healthy teeth and bones.

Eggs

If you are watching your pennies, eggs are one of the least expensive forms of protein. The American Heart Association says normal healthy adults can safely enjoy an egg a day. Go ahead and whip up your favorite scramble, breakfast hash, omelet, or frittata.

Beans

One-half cup of beans contains as much protein as an ounce of broiled steak. Plus, these nutritious nuggets are loaded with fiber to keep you feeling full for hours. Make a batch of mixed bean soup in your crockpot with homemade cornbread. Toss a taco salad and use beans in lieu of chicken or beef or make a homemade hummus like roasted red pepper with chickpeas and serve with pita chips as an appetizer.

Pork

This great and versatile white meat is 31 percent leaner than it was twenty years ago. During a trip to Prague, Budapest, and Vienna we experienced some of the most delectable dinners that contained pork tenderloin. Most of the dinners came with apple dumplings, but I substituted apple stuffing and sautéed apples alongside red cabbage. If you want a show stopper and memorable meal or a change from the traditional holiday dinners, this one is a great choice. You can really get fancy and use a round pork roast with those miniature chef's hats.

Soy

Fifty grams of soy protein daily can lower your cholesterol by as much as 3 percent. Eating soy protein instead of sources of higher fat protein and maintaining a nutritionally balanced diet can be heart healthy. Out of respect for my friends and relatives who are vegan or vegetarian, I am always searching for meals that meet their nutritional preferences.

Lean Beef

Did you know that lean beef has only one more gram of saturated fat than a skinless chicken breast? Many women do not get enough of zinc, iron, and vitamin B12, and lean beef provides all of these. If you have an iron deficiency, a great option is the French dip sandwich, which has thinly sliced roast beef and is served with au jus. Next time you are at your favorite Mexican restaurant, order some beef fajitas, or grill a filet mignon at home.

Protein at Breakfast

Research shows that including a source of protein like an egg or Greek yogurt at breakfast along with a high-fiber grain like whole wheat toast can help you feel full longer and eat less throughout the day. In England it is customary to have soft boiled eggs that sit on adorable egg holder and use your soldiers (toast cut into thin strips) to dip into your eggs. Most children have one with their initials or names engraved, and if you really want to be festive, you can buy tiny toboggans like I did to place on top of the eggs and keep them warm.

In essence, all proteins are not alike, and it is important to be cognizant of this. Protein is built from building blocks called amino acids. Our bodies produce amino acids either from scratch, or by modifying others. A few amino acids (known as the essential amino acids) must come from food. If you are a carnivore, animal sources of protein deliver all of the amino acids that your bodies need. However, other protein sources such as nuts and seeds lack one or more essential amino acids. Therefore, vegetarians and vegans need to be aware of this because they may not eat meat, fish, poultry, eggs, or dairy products. It is essential to consume a variety of protein each day in order to get all the amino acids needed to make new protein. Go ahead and mix it up and have chicken, peanut butter, beans, tofu, eggs, steak, seafood, or pork to make sure you are getting all of the amino acids that your body needs.

Get the Facts on Fats

Many of our patients eat no fat or very minimal amounts, and despite this, some were actually gaining weight. Our dietitians began to see the trend that their fat intake was too low. They weren't satiated since fat sustains us, so they were consuming excessive calories. In my work with childhood obesity and binge eating disorder patients were eating virtually no fat breakfasts (skim milk and cereal with no fat) and lunches (turkey sandwich on whole wheat with mustard and an apple), so they were ravenous after school hours and bingeing. We adjusted their diets to add more fat and protein at breakfast (eggs, Canadian bacon, and whole wheat toast with butter) and lunch (peanut butter and jelly on whole wheat), and they actually began to lose weight. In essence, fats keep us fuller longer and are needed for balanced nutrition.

There is a distinction between healthy and unhealthy fats that needs to be made to have a comprehensive understanding of how fats are beneficial to your food intake. The phrase "healthy fat" usually refers to monounsaturated and polyunsaturated fats, which are considered to be heart healthy, and lower LDL cholesterol, which is the kind that clogs your arteries. Recent studies have shown these fats can benefit insulin and blood sugar levels, decreasing the risk of type 2 diabetes. "Monounsaturated fats are among the healthiest of all fats," Dana Hunnes, PhD, MPH, RD, senior dietician at UCLA Medical Center and adjunct assistant professor at the Fielding School of Public Health, tells SELF magazine, "These are anti-inflammatory, reduce the risk of cardiovascular disease, and are full of healthy nutrients." According to the American Heart Association, trans fats increase your risk of developing heart disease, stroke, and are associated with a higher risk of type 2 diabetes.

The guidance on saturated fat is a little more complicated. Old nutrition research said saturated fat was really bad for your cholesterol levels, but newer information suggests it has a more neutral effect. The topic is very touchy, and the USDA Dietary Guidelines and the American Heart Association still recommend limiting your intake and opting for monounsaturated and polyunsaturated fats instead. Many of the healthy foods below have some saturated fat in them, but it doesn't make up the majority of the fat content and won't negate the positive effects of the healthier fats. The following are some great choices for polyunsaturated and monounsaturated fat:

Avocado

One medium avocado has approximately 23 grams of fat, but it is primarily monounsaturated fat. Plus, a medium avocado contains 40 percent of your daily fiber needs, is naturally sodium and cholesterol-free, and is a good source of lutein, an antioxidant that may protect your vision. Enjoy an avocado on your turkey sandwich or order tableside guacamole dip or try avocado on toast, which is all the rage!

Nuts

Walnuts are one of the best sources of omega-3 fatty acids, specifically alpha linoleic acid, an omega-3 found in plants. A recent study linked a handful per day to lower total cholesterol and LDL cholesterol as well as improved blood vessel functioning. Nuts like pecans, pistachios, cashews, and almonds also pack a lot of healthy fats. Almonds are the richest in vitamin E, and pistachios have lutein and zeaxanthin, carotenoids that are important to eye health. All you need to eat is a 1/4 cup serving per day to reap the benefits. Some varieties are fattier than others, like cashews and macadamia nuts, so be cognizant of your serving sizes. (Nuts have, on average, 45 grams of fat per cup.) You may love eating pistachios because it takes more time to shell them, so you eat slower and control portion size. The peanut (technically a legume) contains monounsaturated fats, but all of its polyunsaturated fats are omega-6s, which evidence suggests may not do us any favors. I love the texture that you get from sunflower seeds and almonds, so I sprinkle them on my berry crisp for a mega dose of healthy fats, protein, and fiber.

An easier way to get all the fatty goodness of nuts may be from a nut or seed butter. Try almond and cashew, or sunflower seed butter, for a plant-based dose of monounsaturated and polyunsaturated fats.

Olives and Olive Oil

One cup of black olives has 15 grams of fat, but again, it is mainly monounsaturated. Plus, no matter what variety of olive you enjoy, they all contain many other beneficial nutrients as well, such as hydroxytyrosol, a phytonutrient that has long been linked to cancer prevention. New research is showing that this phytonutrient may play a role in reducing bone loss as well. And if you have allergies or other inflammatory conditions, olives might be just the snack for you as research suggests that olive extracts function as antihistamines on the cellular level. Even with all these benefits, it is important to be mindful of your serving size as olives can be high in sodium. Stick to 5 large or 10 small olives as the perfect portion. Cooking with olive oil is not only flavorful, but it is full of monounsaturated fats. One tablespoon has 14 grams of fats and 120 calories and can be used as a condiment to dip your bread into or sauté vegetables and meat. So, go ahead and toss some olives onto your Greek salad, pizza, or make a batch of tapenade for as an appetizer.

Salmon and Other Fish

Oily fish like salmon, sardines, or trout are full of omega-3 fatty acids and known to help improve heart health. It's one of the best ways to get essential fat. The American Heart Association recommends eating at least two servings weekly. Ahi tuna also packs a punch on flavor if it is seasoned properly and has a high amount of healthy fats and omega-3s. You may go to your favorite sushi place or create your own tuna tower. Both salmon and tuna should be limited to about 12 ounces (two meals) a week to avoid exposure to mercury that can be found in small amounts in seafood.

Asian Salmon with Susan's Salsa

This lovely Asian salmon dish combines the delicate flavor of fresh salmon and the zing of tropical fruit. Perfect for a summer grill, you serve this alongside grill sweet corn on the cob and Susan's salsa for a fresh and colorful meal. Serves 10–12.

Salmon

3 pounds of salmon filets
2 tablespoons of Dijon mustard
3 tablespoons of light soy sauce
6 tablespoons olive oil
2 teaspoons of minced garlic
½ cup of fresh dill

Susan's Salsa:

1 red onion, diced
4 bell peppers: yellow, red, green, and orange (diced)

1 bunch of cilantro
1 finely chopped jalapeno
1 tablespoon of olive oil
8 ounces of canned tropical fruit (drained)
Sea salt and ground pepper to taste

Prepare and chill the salsa ingredients at least a few hours before you are ready to serve it. Whisk the Dijon mustard, soy sauce, garlic, olive oil, and fresh dill. Pour over the salmon and allow to marinate for one day turning over to insure both sides are marinated. Prepare a mesquite grill and cook the salmon for approximately 4 to 5 minutes on each side. Cover the salmon with foil and allow it to rests for another 5 minutes.

Dark Chocolate

Sometimes when it comes to foods that we perceive as forbidden foods, we may need permission from others or ourselves to eat them. I am giving you permission to enjoy dark chocolate because one ounce of dark chocolate counts as one serving and it contains saturated fat and nutritious nutrients such as vitamins A, B, and E, calcium, iron, potassium, magnesium, and flavonoids (plant-based antioxidants). Aim for a cocoa content of at least 70 percent for the highest levels of flavonoids.

Tofu

Tofu is not as high in fat as the other foods on this list, but it is still a good source of monounsaturated and polyunsaturated fats. A modest, 3-ounce portion of super firm tofu contains 5 to 6 grams of fat and about 1 gram of saturated fat, but this is naturally occurring fat from the soybeans, and tofu is considered a health food for a reason. It's a solid plant-based protein that's low in sodium and provides nearly a quarter of your daily calcium needs.

Eggs

People often think egg whites are a healthier option than whole eggs because they contain less fat, but while it's true that the egg yolk contains some fat, it's also packed with important nutrients. One whole egg contains 5 grams of fat, but only 1.5 grams are saturated. Whole eggs are also a good source of choline (one egg yolk has about 300 micrograms), an important B vitamin that helps regulate the brain, nervous system, and cardiovascular system. As for the cholesterol? The most current research has found that eating cholesterol doesn't raise our blood cholesterol. Research has linked moderate egg consumption to improved heart health.

Parmesan Cheese

I absolutely love parmesan cheese since it has that salty nuttiness, and I keep large containers in my freezer as my "go-to cheese" for cooking. Shards of parmesan or parmesan crisps can be served as an appetizer with cocktails or sprinkled on your favorite Caesar salad. Many people have chosen to omit cheeses that are full of fat like parmesan. Indeed, cheeses do have more saturated fats than plant-based foods, but they (especially Parmesan, which contains 8 grams fat and 5 grams saturated fat per ounce) provide many other nutrients. In fact, parmesan tops the cheese charts in terms of its bone-building calcium content, providing nearly a third of your daily calcium intake. Ounce for ounce, it has more protein than any other food, including meat and eggs.

Fruits and Veggies

My paternal grandfather was a farmer and had the most beautiful garden you can ever imagine. My favorite memories are picking one of his black diamond watermelons and busting it open in the middle of the field and eating it! It was crimson red inside and emerald green on the outside and shaped like a basketball. It was juicy and sweet, and to this day I crave this type of watermelon since it is my favorite fruit! My parents also grew a garden, and we were required to pick the fruits and vegetables, and we thought it was a great way to work on our suntan! It was a golden opportunity to taste test fruits and vegetables as kids, and I think that is why I love cooking and eating them today!

Eating the colors of the rainbow such as vegetables and fruits are a vital part of a balanced and nutritious diet. When you consume these delectable jewels, it is more psychologically pleasing to your palate when your plate contains colorful food. Eating a variety of fruits and vegetables is as critical as the quantity. When was the last time you went to a farmer's market or your favorite grocery store and selected or tried some old favorites and introduced yourself to new ones?

According to a Harvard University study, a diet rich in vegetables and fruits can lower blood pressure, reduce risk of heart disease and stroke, prevent some types of cancer, lower risk of eye and digestive problems, and have a positive effect upon blood sugar, which can help keep appetite in check. Eat a variety of types and colors of produce in order to give your body the mix of nutrients it needs. Try dark leafy greens (kale), brightly colored red (red bell peppers), yellow and orange vegetables and fruits (berries such as blueberries, raspberries, blackberries, or strawberries), and cooked tomatoes.

Roasted Winter Vegetables

Roasted winter vegetables are characteristic of the traditional English meals we have in my husband's native village Sandwich, England. The aromas of the vegetables roasting permeates your kitchen on a cold winter's day! Serves 6.

2 beets
1 bag of parsnips
1 bag of carrots
1 butternut squash
2 sweet potatoes
2 tablespoons of olive oil
1 teaspoon each of sea salt and freshly ground pepper
1 tablespoon each of thyme, parsley, and mint

Peel the beets, parsnips, carrots, sweet potatoes, and butternut squash. Cut into about 1 ½ inch pieces and sprinkle generously with sea salt and pepper. Preheat the oven to 425 degrees. First place the olive oil in the roasting pan and allow the oil to get very hot since this allows the veggies to roast in lieu of steaming. Then toss the vegetables with the olive oil and spread out in a single layer. Stir the veggies occasionally until all sides are roasted and tender. The cooking time may vary depending on your oven temperature, but approximately 20 minutes, or until fork tender. Sprinkle with fresh herbs afterwards.

In summary, my hope is to restore the joy and pleasure of eating. My favorite restaurant is Javier's, which serves gourmet Mexican food, and I have been a patron for over thirty ears. The ambience, friendly waiters, and delectable cuisine make this an amazing dining experience. It is one of my happy places! I am optimistic that we all can learn to have it all when it comes to "having your cake and eating it too." Empowering yourself to see food as a choice whereby you incorporate balanced nutrition and firing the food police will help you overcome emotional eating. As you learn to have your "piece of cake and peace of mind," there are endless possibilities that you will savor in your food journey, and your body esteem will grow exponentially.

Balancing Protein, Carbohydrate, and Fat—(P.C.F)

Why is the P–C–F balance so important?

Eating balanced meals and snacks with a mixture of protein, carbohydrate, and fat will help to regulate and normalize blood sugar throughout the entire day. Eating every three to five hours with a careful combination of carbohydrate, protein, and fat will help regulate your blood sugar level, satisfy your hunger, and reduce the need for overeating or binge eating. Therefore, if your diet is high in carbohydrate, more feedings will be required (4 to 6), and if your diet is higher in fat the fewer feedings per day will be required (3 to 4).

PCF Chart

Food	Effect on Blood Sugar	Time taken to break down to blood sugar
Simple Sugars Sugar, Soft Drinks, Alcohol, Candy, Glucose.	Hour 1 Hour 2 Hour 3 Hour 4 Hour 5	Sugar is broken down very easily, causing a rapid rise and fall in blood sugar (BS). **15–45 minutes**
Complex Carbs Whole Grains, Bread, Fruit, Vegetables, Rice.	Hour 1 Hour 2 Hour 3 Hour 4 Hour 5	Complex carbs (C), are denser so longer to break down than simple sugar causing BS to rise and fall over period of **1–3 hours**
Protein Chicken, Eggs, Milk, Cheese, Red meat, Fish, Tofu, Beans.	Hour 1 Hour 2 Hour 3 Hour 4 Hour 5	Proteins (P) are significantly denser and will take longer to break down to BS. Digestion occurs gradually over a period of **3–5 hours**

Food	Effect on Blood Sugar	Time taken to break down to blood sugar
Fats		=
Butter, Cooking Oils, Salad Dressing, Saturated fats, cream, Ice Cream.	Hour 1 Hour 2 Hour 3 Hour 4 Hour 5	Fats (F) are digested the slowest sustaining a more constant blood sugar over an extended period, from **4–6 hours**

Ideal Feeding Chart

AM PM

Breakfast/Lunch/Snack/Dinner

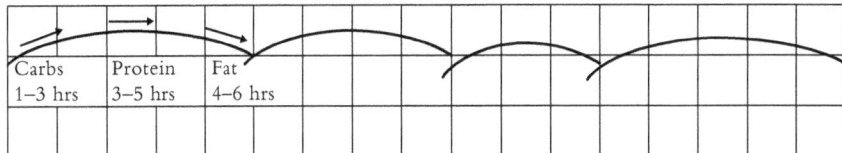

| Carbs | Protein | Fat |
| 1–3 hrs | 3–5 hrs | 4–6 hrs |

Chapter 6
Fashion: Style Icons

"Fashion is about dressing according to what's fashionable. Style is more about being yourself."
—Oscar de la Renta

Meghan Markle's first appearance with Prince Harry after announcing their engagement adhered to the royal dress code yet demonstrated her personal flair. She displayed a sense of style that was similar to the iconic dynasty from her native country with a look reminiscent of the late Carolyn Bessette Kennedy. The fashion statement was a look of sophistication with a neutral color palate. Although the outfits are over two decades apart, the basic elements were similar: a black sweater, a neutral beige midi skirt, as Bessette Kennedy wore her look in 1996 while making an appearance with her husband JFK Jr. outside their Tribeca apartment.

Besette Kennedy was often photographed in a down-to-earth yet chic style. Today, Bessette Kennedy's style is nearly as iconic as that of her mother-in-law, Jackie Kennedy. All three of these women have one common denominator in their style: it is classic and timeless. Through the ages not only have they become style icons that inspire a generation of women, but they dress beautifully and own their style with how they carry themselves, accentuated by an air of confidence.

This chapter will help you capture your own sense of style and build a wardrobe that will not only reflect your personality but flatter your figure. You will learn techniques on how to exude body esteem by the manner in which you dress and walk out to meet the world each day.

Calendar Girls

During a visit to England I noticed a calendar with middle aged women practically nude and when I asked my mother in law, Olive what it was she replied, "Oh those are the calendar girls!" Olive was a shy English lady, so I was surprised to hear that the Women's Institute, which she had been a member of, was raising money for one of the calendar girl's husband who had cancer. One of the calendar girls set at the piano nude, and all you could see was her butt crack, and another one held two large cupcakes in front of her breasts. Years later this was made into a movie and a play I saw with my family in Canterbury! It was hysterical! What I found most fascinating is that the calendar girls were like many of us in that there was some anxiety about posing nude even for a great cause!

I want my legacy to be that I helped others overcome body shame. It manifests itself in so many areas of our lives, and it seems more prevalent when we are shopping for clothes (i.e., swimsuit season) or cleaning out our closets. I am not suggesting that we need to strip down for a photo shoot, but I do want you to have confidence and enjoy your body. The fashion quotient (FQ) will help you overcome insecurities as you learn to style your clothing. There is no shame in showcasing your silhouette, so let's begin in the dressing room where a lack of confidence seems to play out the most!

Retail Therapy

Have you literally ever shopped until you dropped? Retail therapy is a method that is often used to manage stress. Yet it can also be a pleasurable experience to go shopping and find some treasures. The pendulum for shopping can actually swing both ways if we are uncomfortable in our own body. You may find that you compulsively shop for the perfect garments to help you feel better about your body and appearance. Perhaps you avoid shopping altogether because you fear you have gone up a size and are afraid to try on the clothes in your closet that may no longer fit. You may feel that you have limited options when it comes to the clothes that fit your body properly. Sometimes it seems easier to hang out in your pajamas or yoga pants! You may become irritable or sad, and you are convinced you have nothing to wear, yet you are reluctant to shop for anything new. Getting dressed does not have to be an excruciating task! Let's break this self-defeating cycle so that you can become fashion forward and achieve body esteem.

Furthermore, you may have left behind much of your self-care and beauty regimen you used to implement on a daily basis. In essence, body dissatisfaction has a major impact on your fashion and sense of style. This chapter will give you the tools you need to have a "passion for fashion" and show you how to use fashion as your ally to improve your body esteem. Although your fashion quotient (FQ) is only one aspect of your body esteem quotient, I believe it is an important one. Fashion can foster a sense of appreciation when it comes to your appearance and body image.

Your fashion quotient (FQ) can serve you well in terms of camouflaging your perceived figure flaws (buttocks) and accentuating your assets (defined waistline). If your body shape has changed, fashion can be used to enhance or minimize these changes. In other body quotients, we are investing in what concerns us internally by improving our nutrition and becoming more psychologically introspective. And, the exercise quotient is a nice bridge between the internal and external because internal muscle development affects the external look of how clothes fit us. Although it is important to address all of the quotients, the fashion quotient can often have immediate and positive results. Think of the many makeovers that you've seen in media and magazines that play up your delicate features such as cheekbones. You can see the participant blossom right in front of your eyes. True, any temporary state needs a sustainable path to keep it going, but increasing your fashion quotient can give you a lift while you work to build your other quotients and overall body esteem.

FQ: Fashion is only one aspect of improving your body esteem and the other building blocks such as PQ, NQ, and EQ must be addressed as well. Your FQ may provide more immediate results and keep you motivated as you work on the other quotients, which all complement each other and enhance the whole.

Fashion Quotient Assessment

1. Your personal style should
   a. Copy celebrities
   b. Follow only recent trends
   c. Reflect your autonomy
   d. Must be done only with a stylist

2. When building your sense of style and wardrobe one should
   a. Consider your body type
   b. Adhere to your budget
   c. Learn to trust your judgement
   d. All of the above

3. One of the most important rules to follow in styling your wardrobe is
   a. Ask the salesperson how you look
   b. Bring a friend along to help you make good choices
   c. Always defer to others for their approval
   d. Learn to validate your self-esteem and body image

4. What factors into flattering your body type
   a. Color tones and hues
   b. Color blocking
   c. Well-tailored clothing
   d. All of the above

5. Which of the following are not essential wardrobe pieces?
   a. Jeans
   b. Blazers
   c. Wedge shoes
   d. undergarments

6. When shopping for a swimsuit you should
    a. Choose the one that you love the most
    b. Consider trends for that season
    c. Be cognizant that swimsuits are usually a few sizes larger
    d. Bring your significant other to help you choose

7. Couture clothing is
    a. A must when building your wardrobe
    b. Is more expensive but typically fits your body better
    c. Always needs to be tailored
    d. Less expensive

8. When seeking out a tailor it is best to
    a. Find out their educational background and credentials
    b. Have your new clothes tailored at the store that you purchased them
    c. Request the fee beforehand
    d. All of the above

9. Compulsive Buying Disorder
    a. Only pertains to what you actually purchase
    b. Manifests itself typically in adulthood
    c. Can lead to chronic debt or bankrupt and have a negative impact on relationship
    d. Does not have a correlation to body image

10. How does your fashion quotient impact your nutrition quotient, exercise quotient, and psychological quotient?
    a. Your fashion quotient is only one aspect of your four quotients and fosters better body image.
    b. It is the most important and critical quotient.
    c. It cannot be used until you master your other quotients.
    d. None of the above

11. As you improve your fashion quotient, it is essential to
    a. Follow the systematic methodology to eliminate or alter clothes that no longer fit
    b. Learn to be patient with yourself and trust your judgement
    c. Not seek out the advice or validation from others
    d. All of the above

12. Which emotions impact your fashion quotient and self-esteem?
    a. Anxiety
    b. Depression
    c. Stress
    d. All of the above

13. How does one began to be in touch with their own body and choose a wardrobe?
    a. Acknowledge an accurate depiction of your body
    b. Be cognizant that various sizes fit everyone differently
    c. Learn to accentuate your assets and camouflage your body dissatisfaction
    d. All of the above

14. Fashion quotient can be improved by
    a. Educating yourself
    b. Only attending fashion week in New York
    c. Purchasing the most expensive designer clothes
    d. Wearing less expensive clothes

15. What is the biggest fashion faux pas?
    a. Wearing oversized clothing or clothes skin tight
    b. Wearing inexpensive clothes
    c. Wearing only bold colors
    d. Wearing Spanx or undergarments

You can find the answers at www.bodyesteem.com

Curate Your Own Closet (#CYOC)

As the body changes, shopping for new clothes or pursuing alterations with a tailor is important to staying in the present and appreciating your body as it is—even if you are actively working to change some things about it. As your shape or size changes, the important focus is to only have clothing that fits your body as it currently is. I know many of us keep a closet full of several sizes, which is fine as long as the reason for different sizes is to accommodate small fluctuations. But hanging on to clothing that is now too large to wear is sending your brain a message that you expect to fail and regain your weight and you better have some clothes saved "just in case." The other end of the spectrum is just as unsettling. When you keep clothing that is now too small, it says that you are hanging on to a "better" size for you, which also sends the message that you are unhappy with your body.

Jenna Bush-Hager wrote a letter to her daughters, Mila and Poppy, about lessons she learned from her parents: "They taught me that who I am is more important than how I look. And that if I radiate love, kindness, and empathy, I can bring some light to this dark world (and isn't that better than being a size zero?)." Appreciate and enjoy your body at your current size. Generally speaking, the variance in clothing sizes is typically two to three sizes. If you want to change something, great. But wearing clothes that fit you and feeling that you look good every day bolsters your self-confidence and brings you out of a cycle of waiting for something else to happen, whether the "coming" change is perceived as a positive or a negative. Otherwise, there is a tendency to feel inadequate or to continue to have an unrealistic view of your body. You won't have to encounter any triggers of guilt or dismay as you avoid certain clothes or push others to the background "just in case." Be aware that by having access to only clothes that fit you, there is no emotional minefield every time you open your closet door or paw through a drawer.

Sorting through all of your clothes can unearth lots of hidden gems. A therapeutic activity is to curate your own closet (#CYOC). Weight variances happen for most women, whether it be weight gain due to having a baby, your monthly cycle, or perimenopause, and later, menopause. While our weight may be somewhat consistent, it often shifts to other body regions such when you notice that you've begun to carry more weight in your lower body (i.e., stomach, legs, hips, and thighs) and later in life it may be in the upper part (i.e., breasts, waist, arms, and back). It is not uncommon for a woman to gain or shift their lower body weight to their upper body during perimenopause and menopause. Now, this is where fashion can really become the equalizer. A secret weapon is to wear darker clothes for your upper body such as a beautiful berry silk blouse, which will serve to minimize your torso and arms. Or, wear darker pants or skirts if your lower body needs that fix. Even Cindy Crawford acknowledged that her weight has shifted to other places as she has aged gracefully. Physiologically speaking, it is completely unrealistic to think that you will maintain the same weight and body composition throughout your lifespan. To embrace that fact and use your closet as a strategy is a proactive body strategy.

Similar to a curator of a museum, you are the curator of your own closet (#CYOC), and this act will actually empower you to be in control of your collection of clothing. Therefore, educate yourself and plan ahead for the times that you experience weight fluctuations. During these times, reorganizing your closet into sizes that may have more generous fabric and focusing on accessories like those lovely red patent stilettos and matching clutch builds body positivity. The actual act of decluttering your closet and systematically reorganizing it into a range of sizes that adapt to your weight changes introduces body esteem. Furthermore, holding onto clothes that are excessively large or small may actually weigh you down literally and figuratively speaking.

Curating your own closet (#CYOC) may bring up emotions, but I am optimistic that it will allow you to move forward. I am confident in this process because I have guided my patients through this cathartic experience. If you have suffered from a formal eating disorder, as you recover, it is actually therapeutic to donate your skinny jeans to charity. If you have been obese and lost a significant amount of weight, discard your larger sizes of clothing because the mental adjustment takes time to acclimate to your new size.

On the bright side, you are making room for new articles of clothing and embracing being a woman and not wearing preteen sizes that are not meant to last you a lifetime. Donating your clothes to charities helps other women have a new wardrobe and a new lease on life to jumpstart their body esteem. And what you now have curated are outfits you know will fit you and look good on you and that you feel good wearing! Sorting through and cleaning out your closet can help you mix and match outfits that you forgot you even had.

Likewise, curating your closet is similar to a museum having a special exhibit with a small section of your closet devoted to the times when you may be bloated due to ovulation or your menses. These clothes may not be as fitted as your other garments, but can be just as chic and might feature a pop of color, such as a classic poncho, a marigold maxi dress, or a designer tunic. Similar to an exhibit being displayed, you only wear these garments for short bursts of time to accommodate these normal bodily changes.

Learn to use the fashion quotient by taking inventory of your closet and your personal needs in a systematic and methodical manner. Follow the fashion advice so that you too can become the curator of your closet:

CYOC#1: Visualize this process as if you are a buyer in a retail store and you are taking inventory and replenishing merchandise. Independently remove each category of clothing outside of your closet to formulate a clearer picture of your wardrobe. Start with your shapewear and move to each section from blazers, jeans, and dresses to accessories. If any of the merchandise is too worn, dated, or cannot be altered to fit your body, discard it. Carefully pin and/or take pictures of each category and record where you are lacking in your wardrobe (sandals for summer) and strategically plan to shop for these items as a priority before you make other purchases. If you have plenty of storage space, you may want to separate your clothes by seasons to improve organization in your closet.

CYOC #2: Once you have completed your documentation, review your Pinterest and/or pictures in a quiet place outside your closet to determine which ones fit your body properly. Immediately remove ones that are unrealistic to wear (i.e., maternity clothes if you are not planning to have another baby). Assess the garments that can be altered by a tailor (i.e., inserting fabric in the waistline or taking darts out of a blazer or blouse). Ask yourself if you can fit into them within the next year (i.e., recovering from surgery), and if the answer is no, donate them to charity or take them to a resale shop. Meanwhile, for the ones that you plan to keep, remove the much smaller or larger sizes and store them outside of your closet.

CYOC #3: Now comes the fun part! You may find that you need or prefer only a few key items for refreshers for your wardrobe (i.e., a rose gold leather jacket). Look at all of the trends and find some items that work well for your body type and allow yourself to invest in a stylistic item (i.e., embroidered butterfly wing ballet flats). Allow yourself a budget for spending and dedicate the amount you can actually afford. Now take yourself on a shopping spree where you actually give yourself permission to enjoy the experience without having buyer's remorse. Make the experience more memorable by going out to lunch or afternoon tea.

FQ: The first step in improving your fashion quotient is to take a systematic inventory of your closet by assessing what specific garments or accessories you need. Secondly, identify which are interchangeable such as garments that can work with several pieces in your wardrobe like a black velvet blazer and carefully pin information for your planned shopping experience.

No More Fashion Faux Paus

There are fashion faux pas that are missteps, but there is no need to be so critical of yourself or of one another. It is important to approach fashion with a spirit of adventure and self-discovery. Shaming or second-guessing yourself is going to keep you locked in to what you already know and have already experienced that has been less than what you now want. Free yourself from your own inner critic. More importantly body shaming yourself because you believe that you do not look good in one style or a particular color is counterproductive. The key is to experiment, experience, see what it feels like, and choose what you want to embrace and integrate into your style. Even accepting that you are going to wear a fun style for a season gives you permission to try something new. Most importantly, it keeps you moving forward, rather than being affected by the past.

Allow yourself to gradually master your sense of style by not looking to others for validation. If you have any fashion police in your life or you are your own fashion police, fire them or yourself immediately. Your fashion quotient will not improve if you are allowing others to be critical of your attire or body, and your own self-punitive thoughts only negate your efforts. When was the last time that you asked someone "Do you think I look fat in this outfit?" Stop asking others what they think about your style of dress. It is best to not set yourself up for criticism, and it certainly does you no good when it comes to your fashion quotient or psychological quotient. You do not need anyone to validate your body or sense of style.

FQ: Fire the fashion police and stop being so self-critical about your style because you will make side-steps along the way. Do not seek validation or feedback from others in regard to your appearance, style, or body.

Know Thy Own Body

There is only one you, and it is important that you "know thy own body" before you establish your signature style. At this stage you may not even know what your signature style is when it comes to fashion because it often evolves serendipitously. One method of how to develop this is to start outside the world of fashion and look at your preferences in art, music, and décor. You may prefer the clean lines and structure of modern and contemporary art and asymmetric and edgy designs appeal to you. Perhaps your eye is drawn to French Impressionists such as Monet because the color palettes he painted captured the sunlight. When it comes to décor you gravitate towards eclecticism and mix and match antiques with more modern and contemporary accents. The key is to find inspiration for your sense of style via your surroundings and experiences.

As you discover your signature style, it is important to embrace your body type, accentuate your assets, and minimize your perceived figure flaws—also known as what most bothers you. My assets are my dimples, authentic perky busts, narrow hips, toned legs from ballroom dancing, twin toes that are grown together I named "Tootsie," and a birthmark called "Bertha!" My figure flaws are having a short waist and a flat butt! I could buy a butt bra to have a fuller butt, but one bra is enough! Besides, I have learned to dress where I emphasize my strengths (i.e., sheath dresses and jumpsuits) and downplay my weaknesses (i.e., monochromatic colors like midnight blue with various textures that lengthen my torso).

I love to use scarves such as a bright paisley or equestrian print and tie them on my handbags to offset the monochromatic tones and jewelry (a stack of tricolor bangles and multicolored drop earrings) that suit my personality! My smile is free, and the best asset that I have is to keep smiling to show off my dimples! Of course, I throw in some whimsical pieces like my piano clutch that represents my passion for being a pianist! Take a moment and establish your body type, and once you do this activity it will make fashion choices much easier!

Identify what will not change with your body with exercise, nutrition, and wishful thinking. There are specific regions that may not respond with weight loss or gain: short waist, long waist, and round, narrow or heart shaped face, or muscular calves. Why beat yourself up when you have no control over some of these issues? The good news is that your fashion quotient can help you find a formula to feel better about these bodily areas. I do not believe in labeling your body type (i.e., pear shape) because it can be self-deprecating. The fashion formula will clearly delineate some guidelines that accentuate your assets and camouflage specific regions where you have body dissatisfaction. If there is a tendency to carry your weight in your midsection, the objective is to counteract this by creating lines that minimize this body region. Invest in undergarments such as Spanx that give you a sleek and smooth silhouette. Building structure into your style is essential since shapeless blouses or clothing are not flattering.

My clinical impressions are that learning to let go of specific body regions that may not respond to healthy nutrition and exercise is challenging but obtainable and necessary to foster body esteem. Fortunately, your fashion quotient can serve as your secret weapon to help you embrace this process and to not be so preoccupied with something that you cannot change.

FQ: Identify and embrace the body regions that may not change with exercise and nutrition. Utilize your fashion quotient to help you through this process.

Back to Basics

There are timeless pieces in your wardrobe that will carry you through the years, and every woman may want to invest in these to avoid feeling "I can't find anything to wear in my closet!" If you build a wardrobe based on "back to the basics," you will always find what you are looking for in your closet. "Rome wasn't built in a day," and the same applies to your wardrobe. Be patient with yourself and methodically prioritize which aspects of your wardrobe need to be built first (business or casual). The following are the basics that one may consider incorporating into their wardrobe:

- Shapewear and undergarments
- Workout clothes
- Crisp white blouse
- Silk and cotton shirts in your color pallets
- Jeans that go from daytime to evening
- Boots (ankle and knee high) in suede or leather
- Stilettoes (beige and black)
- Blazers in colors that coordinate with your wardrobe (amethyst)
- Skirts (classic pencil)
- Dresses in your favorite hues
- A little black dress
- A stunning cocktail dress
- An elegant long evening gown
- A luxurious coat with a scarf and gloves
- Sweaters and sweater sets in soft cashmere
- Tailored dress pants
- A sexy swimsuit, cover-up or sarong, and sandals
- Eccentric sneakers in silver, gold, or rose gold for dressing up or down
- Accessories such as jewelry, scarves, and cravats

Be Your Own Stylist (#BYOS)

I have confidence in your ability to be your own stylist (#BYOS). Utilize your creative temperament and incorporate these fundamental pieces interchangeably so it expands your wardrobe. Pull out each of the garments above and pin or take photos of the various ways you can create more outfits. Start with your jeans and add every blouse and sweater, and pair them with different shoes and boots. Next move to your skirts and blazers and implement the same technique by mixing and matching. Utilize your accessories by adding scarves, bracelets, statement pieces, and so on for as many different looks as you can imagine. The possibilities are endless, but remember that "less is more," and if your accessories are excessive, remove some pieces until you find the look you are after. Along the way challenge yourself to coordinate as many pieces of your basic wardrobe as possible. The objective is to learn to trust your judgement, style your own clothes, and feel empowered.

In the event that you find that it is too challenging to be your own stylist (#BYOS), you may seek out a personal stylist to artistically create your wardrobe. However, style books and magazines provide a wealth of information on style and are a great resource and guide. There are myriad shapes and silhouettes in the marketplace, and trends evolve daily, but I am confident you can learn to navigate through this process. Jennifer Aniston once said that she does not purchase or follow trends, which is a good rule of thumb. If you find designers or trends that work well, only introduce new ones if the style flatters your figure.

A fashion prescription for your body does not have to be hard-and-fast rules but a formula that you follow. This formula requires you to be comfortable in your clothing and wear only styles that build self-confidence and body esteem. If you have concerns about your silhouette, invest in quality undergarments and body shapers that give you a sleek and smooth silhouette.

This task may sound daunting, but implementing the style that works best for you is easier than you may think. It requires knowledge, experience, and most of all, learning to trust your judgement. Under no circumstances are you to ask others to validate your body image, whether it be a salesperson, spouse, friend, or relative. You live in this body and know it best and the goal is to learn to increase your fashion quotient (FQ) and validate yourself.

FQ: Once you acquire adequate knowledge about how to improve your fashion quotient, do not seek out validation from others regarding your body and style of dress.

Personal Style: A Fashion Collage (#FC)

A fashion collage (#FC) can spur on ideas to help you define your signature style, which can be very exciting! Go through your closet and select your favorite articles of clothing and record the reasons why you gravitate to these pieces in your wardrobe (i.e., comfort, color, great fit, etc.). Second, look at fashion magazines, apps, and research online clothing, and select the styles that you desire the most. Utilize Pinterest to organize the specific styles that inspire you and your personal style that work for your body type. You may begin to see a pattern in terms of your preferences (i.e., halter jumpsuits with stilettoes or bohemian chic with flowing skirts and a denim jacket and boots).

The most important part of this exercise is to develop your signature style and select clothing that actually works for you. It is essential to approach this exercise where you are not mimicking someone else's style such as a friend or celebrity. Many adolescents and young adults often adopt their friends' or peers' style in fashion because they want to fit in. Most people attempt to pursue their taste in fashion based on others. You may copy Blake Lively, but you are your own unique person and express your autonomy via your fashion collage (#FC). When it comes to your personal style, become your own trend setter

Flaunt Your Favorite Features (#FYFF)

Focus on flaunting your favorite features (#FYFF) in regard to your body! Sometimes we become so preoccupied with our figure flaws that we lose sight of our body regions that we need to showcase. Here are a few fashion tips that will help you learn to flaunt your favorite features or give the illusion that you can profile them:

Rearview Mirror: If your derriere is an asset, then by all means highlight it with a pencil skirt that hugs your buttocks for a classic and timeless look. Perhaps skinny jeans will hug your backside in all of the right places or silk pants skim you beautifully as the fabric drapes over your butt, and a high-heeled pair of shoes gives you just the lift you are looking for!

Get Waisted: The wrap dress was initially designed by Diane von Furstenberg in the seventies, and not only is it the ultimate garment in elegance and sophistication, it is one of the most infallible garments for a woman's body. The wrap dress is waist-centric and defines the smallest point on the body with a fabric tied belt, making it one of the best options for "getting waisted." Accentuate your waist with various belts like chain belts, thin or thick belts, or a rope belt. Similar to the peplum style, fit and flare silhouettes feature demure drop waists and flirty hemlines to accentuate the body at the waistline. A blazer that is well-tailored with a nipped waist and maximum darting and seaming creates a structured silhouette that can work miracles for a feminine feature.

Show Some Leg: Skirts and dresses in all lengths will show your lovely legs! A skirt with a slit profiles toned legs! Don't hide your gazelle-like legs but opt for short hem lines like a leather mini skirt when appropriate. Trending sneakers, ballet flats, and stilettoes all work for long legs. Cropped jackets and cigarette trousers both offer the illusion of longer legs. Lengthen your leg line with monochromatic colors where your shoes match your pants (i.e., emerald green pants with emerald suede boots). Nude stilettoes or wedges give the fashion illusion that you have beautiful long legs!

Belly Buttons: If you have a flat stomach, flaunt it with mid-length tops or a bikini that shows your belly button! Selecting tops where the seams are on the outside edge of your shoulder gives the illusion that your stomach is flatter. Shop for tops that have draping across the belly because this can minimize the stomach region and provide support. Incorporate your undergarments such as Spanx with a camisole or long tank bra that gives you a smooth silhouette. Empire-waist dresses and tops and tunics camouflage the stomach area. Avoid wearing clothes too tight or too loose since this can make the stomach look larger. A-line dresses and wide pants are another secret weapon to minimize the stomach region.

Sizesism

My late mother- and father-in-law gave me a lovely English riding jacket for our first Christmas together in England, and my father-in-law said every lassie (woman) needs a proper one! My father-in-law had a wonderful British humor, and he would greet me by saying, "How's my favorite daughter-in-law from America?" I would laugh and say, "Peter, I am your only daughter-in-law and the only American in the family!" I love wearing it with jodhpurs and English riding boots and like to think of myself as an English rose, but I still do not have the accent down! I adore this riding jacket because it has such sentimental feelings attached to this memory.

Generally speaking, most European designs are larger in sizes than American designs. Historically, retail stores custom made your clothing: you could choose your own fabric, and measurements were taken along with several fittings. There are still designers that customize clothing for clients; if this is economically feasible, it is a viable option. The aforementioned options are still available, and they may minimize issues with sizeism. Meanwhile, the majority of us shop online with free delivery and returns or in retail/boutique stores.

You may not realize that designers work with their own fit and cut garments in their own particular version of a typical size. This is why you may need to try on at least a couple of different sizes when shopping across brands or designers. Most of the couture designs are smaller sizes, and there is not as much room for alterations. It appears counterintuitive, but as I have done with my patients for years, let's go on an imaginary shopping spree to confirm this theory. The first stop is at The Gap where you may actually be a size 8. You walk into Escada (a German design), and you may be a size 10 or 12 because European clothing lines are generally one to two sizes larger. Let's pop into Ralph Lauren where you may be a size 8 or 10. If you hold up all of the garments you will see that the waist size and the jacket size match one another in diameter.

FQ: Do not allow the variance in sizes of clothing be a deterrent for not purchasing merchandise but educate yourself on how designers cut their fashion designs.

A Rainbow of Colors

Now that we've reconciled the great debate over what fits you, let's move on to the colors you enjoy and look best in. You want to find the colors that work for your skin tone and body. The colors for each season change as much as the seasons themselves. And fashion revolves around change, so every season has a popular color. Remember that you are choosing for yourself, so if the color of the season is a hue that you don't feel comfortable wearing like peacock, incorporate it into your accessories such as a clutch or tote. Did you know that burgundy, navy, berry, emerald green, charcoal gray, and royal blue have all been at one time or another dubbed as the new black? Most of us have pieces of clothing that are black, which is very flattering for the majority of us. However, do not be afraid to try colors that may work just as well.

Experiment with color to enhance your mood. Analogous to paint in a room one chooses colors to either make the room look smaller or larger. You may paint your room emerald green for a cozier effect or periwinkle, a pastel that will enlarge the room. Be cognizant of the fact that light and bright colors will accentuate, and dark colors will minimize specific body regions. Color blocking is a great way to minimize specific body areas such as a cobalt blue sheath dress with black-colored panels on both sides of your body that creates a shadow effect where your body will look narrower and your waist will be visually cinched, creating the look of an hourglass figure. Your hips and legs will look more slender due to the strategic placement of the color blocking. Make note of the colors that you feel best in and that lift your spirit. It is paramount to remember that just because you like a color does not mean it will work well in your color palette for your wardrobe. When considering your color palette and whether you should implement it into your wardrobe consider the following:

- BASIC COLORS: These are colors you will wear frequently and are primarily in your fundamental garments like pants, jackets, coats, raincoat, and shoes.
- NEUTRALS: These are colors that complement your basic colors well such as tops, blouses, tanks, shirts, camisoles, and cardigans.

- ACCENT COLORS: Accent colors can be incorporated into your wardrobe and are typically colors you find in your accessories such as handbags, jewelry, some shoes, and scarves.
- OCCASIONAL COLORS: Colors that you gravitate to when you are looking for that power suit or want to express your more whimsical and playful side.

Fabrics: Soft and Cozy

Fabric is your friend. It often determines how the garment hangs and navigates around our curves. Fabric is different from fit, and many people forget that fabric can be used as an ally in helping us define our look. The basic fabrics to choose are cashmere, cotton, wool, silk, and synthetics. The priority when choosing a fabric is to make certain it is appropriate for daytime versus evening wear. Many evites, or invitations address the specific attire such as cocktail or business. Some fabrics are versatile enough that they can take you from day into evening like silk, velvet, or even lace. I have worn a burgundy velvet Ralph Lauren pantsuit or a navy lace dress for charity luncheons when the attire is not specified. If you are dressing as a professional, it is imperative to follow the dress code for that particular company since most have a business dress code. Comfort is key, and the fabric on your skin needs to feel soft and cozy, but if your clothes are not comfortable or you are allergic to certain fabrics like cashmere or wool, you are not going to feel your best. Less expensive fabrics tend to not be as flattering as more expensive ones. Sweater sets that contain silk are also comfortable, can be dressed up or down, and are great for traveling since they do not wrinkle easily. Obviously cotton, the "fabric of our life," and jeans in a myriad of colors are also comfy!

Dress Code Concepts

The dress code in general has become more casual over the years. Take a look at the new rules:

- Extremely Casual which means there are simply no rules and if you are attending a party the guests can wear ripped jeans, shorts, or whatever they prefer (i.e., blue jean shorts, tank tops of your favorite band or business logo, silver hoop earrings, and sandals).

- Very Casual is where you can still dress in a relaxed manner with faded jeans, sneakers, etc., and this is a great opportunity to express your own individual style. Some businesses and parties welcome this style of dress (i.e., faded jeans, embellished sweater, and multicolored wedges).

- Jeans Casual is a trend that some businesses are endorsing where you can still wear jeans, but they need to be more polished and not ripped, faded, or too worn. Flip flops, slippers, and sneakers are not acceptable under this code (i.e., well-tailored dark denim designer jeans with an ivory cashmere sweater or ombre pullover top, gold love knot earrings, or your initial necklace in rose gold, and brown suede ankle boots).

- Slacks Casual is where the focal point is on slacks and one wears a more polished look with crisp fabrics and looks more presentable to colleagues and coworkers. Heels and leather shoes that up your game are highly recommended (i.e., black pencil pants with a crisp white poplin shirt and an emerald green cardigan, scarf or cravat or opera length pearls, and black patent mules or heels).

- Business is whereby the employee is required to wear business attire, which means business suits with ties and oxford dress shirts and dress shoes for men. Women need to wear coordinated styles with a matching blazer and pants/skirt and heels that are not too high are suggested. Law offices, Wall Street, and more industrialized companies require this due to client interaction and an attempt to portray a professional image (a pinstripe gray and lavender pantsuit with a lavender silk blouse, a statement piece necklace or black pearl earrings, and gray sling back heels).

- Cocktail attire is typically where the ladies can wear short cocktail dresses, or a tailored tuxedo suit and the men generally wear suits with a tie or a sports jacket over tailored pants or a sweater without a tie. Other great options are a teal ruched satin cocktail dress or off the shoulder or sweetheart neckline in black lace or red velvet.

- Black Tie is a formal event such as a gala or wedding, and this is a Cinderella moment for women where they can wear a formal ball gown with stiletto shoes (i.e., a stunning beautiful hot pink sequined gown, chandelier or diamond earrings, and strappy metallic sandals or an exquisite sky blue satin mermaid ball gown), and men are required to wear tuxedos only.

My philosophy when it comes to building your personal style that works well in your wardrobe is "more is less." I purchased a red cashmere coat years ago, and I still wear and love this coat. Invest in quality clothing and ask yourself the question: "Will I wear this for years to come?" and if the answer is yes, then it may be worth the investment versus buying trends for one season. It is important to make sure if you invest in an expensive garment that it can be altered as your body may change over the years. Heavy tweeds and wools or chunky cable sweaters may make you look larger than you actually are, so choose wisely.

Foundation and Basics

Hoda and Kathy Lee on the *Today* show have great fun talking about their shapewear alerts (when their undergarments are showing). We all come in different shapes and sizes, and shapewear is essential because it improves our fashion quotient. It is the basic foundation of our wardrobe and provides a smooth silhouette for your body as well as a secret weapon for your figure flaws. But, being comfortable in your clothes is also important, so my suggestion is to find a brand of shapewear that is comfortable but also adds basic support. If you haven't tried on any shapewear in recent years, fabrics have also benefitted from technology, and shapewear is now more breathable and more flexible than it was even just a few years ago. It is well worth an afternoon of shopping to find a brand and some pieces you like. Take a few of your favorite pieces of clothing along to wear over the shapewear to get the intended effect. We're not meant to see shapewear, as Kathy Lee and Hoda will tell you. So, the real test is how your clothing looks over it and how you feel while wearing it. And be sure to sit in any shapewear you consider.

If you are genetically predisposed to specific body regions where you carry your weight, shapewear will minimize these areas. You may have a tendency as you age to have back adipose tissue (back fat), which is difficult to reduce. Sometimes it does not respond well to diet and exercise, but utilizing the right shapewear can be extremely helpful. The right camisole or bra can make the appearance of this fat disappear under your clothing. Spend some type in a reputable lingerie department and have your bra size assessed at least once a year and select foundations that meet your personal body needs. It will make a big difference in how you see yourself in the mirror.

Jeans

Jeans are a frequent favorite for most women. They are comfortable, uncontrived, and sexy if you find the right pair that fits you like a glove. We now see that many women have a mini-wardrobe of jeans that run the gamut in style from weekend casual or work appropriate to nighttime sexy. If you have to try on a gazillion pairs of jeans until you find the style that suits your body, it may be worth it. Some of the most popular jean cuts are trouser, boot cut, boyfriend, girlfriend, straight leg, low-waist, high-waist, and skinny. The beauty of having jeans in your wardrobe is that you can take them from daytime into evening by changing your boots to strappy sandals and adding a sequined or silk blouse. Because of their versatility, traveling with jeans in your wardrobe can certainly give you more room in your suitcase if you plan ahead and pack accordingly.

There are a few fundamental style tips to be cognizant of when purchasing jeans. Similar to choosing colors that work for you, the darker the denim the more slimming effect. The jeans that stretch are going to provide great comfort and fit. If you have a short waist and long legs, gravitate towards jeans that are low rise and elongate your torso. If you are petite it is best to select jeans that adapt to your small frame and set at your waist. Curvy women look fantastic in jeans, and stretch jeans works beautifully to show case your derriere and hips.

Tops

In general, blouses that are the most flattering for everyone are the long sleeve ones that have a high armhole and are tapered and fitted at the wrist since this provides comfort and ease as well as style. Some women may not feel as trendy in this type of blouse, so they opt for necklines that are a cold shoulder, halter, boat, round, or deep V neckline, all of which are great options. Jazz up your blouse by inserting whimsical cuff

links in lieu of buttons. I love how French cuffs give a blouse a more polished and sophisticated look and ties at the wrist add a feminine touch.
Some women are conscious of their upper arms as they age and generally
speaking long sleeve, bracelet sleeve, or three-fourths length work well. If
you have large breasts, you may want to avoid ruffles because they make
breasts appear even larger. By and large the collar shape of a blouse is
important, and the opposite shape of your face works best. When it comes
to the neckline, whether it be a sweater, blouse, or top, the more open
your neckline the more it will elongate your neck, so V-necks or a scoop
neckline are great options.

Swimsuits

Shopping for a swimsuit does not have to be stressful! It is essential to
remember that swimsuits usually are a size or two above our other clothing, and many of us are simply wearing the wrong size. Try styles that
are sold as separates that can accommodate a difference in your top and
bottom size. It might be helpful to know that most of us are not the exact
same size on top as we are on the bottom. If this is the case for you, do
not try to squeeze yourself into a suit when you know the top and bottom
need different sizes.

Years ago, I went shopping for a swimsuit and selected a halter shape
tankini in navy with red trim. I surveyed myself in the mirror and did a
mental checklist for my body type (i.e., elongated my waistline with the
V shape and navy-blue monochromatic color tone). The salesperson said
without my elicitation that she did not think it did anything for my body.
For the first time in many years I elected to not buy the swimsuit based on
her feedback. After reflecting on the conversation, I returned the next day
and purchased the swimsuit. It happens to be my favorite swimsuit ever,
and I feel fit and fabulous in it!

There is a specific fashion formula that you can follow when shopping
for a swimsuit. It is important to note that not all swimsuits are going to
flatter our body, and most only last for a few seasons. Make a decision in
advance about what kind of swimsuit you are going to wear (two-piece,
one piece, boy cut) and consider your body regions such as your legs and
beautiful breasts. Make a mental note of what might have changed since

you last bought a swimsuit. As you are shopping, consider swimsuits that will highlight your assets and minimize your weaknesses: A one-piece swimsuit that has ruching and a darker color to minimize your midsection, a French cut that shows off your legs, and a cup size that complements your décolletage would work beautifully. If you have a long torso, a defined waistline, and small breasts, you may want to try on a bikini to profile your body. If you carry your weight in the lower part of the body, select darker colors such as burgundy or navy and lighter colors for the top.

Accessories

Styling your accessories can be great fun! You can play around with bracelets and mix and match them or some lovely necklaces in various lengths. Whether you are investing in a statement piece or fine jewelry, it is important to remember that shapes and styles must be considered. There are many methods for selecting your jewelry, such as skin tone, but I believe the best way is to determine the shape of your face. Round faces are essentially a perfect circle, so earrings that are long and angled compliment this shape. Oval faces are generally one-and-a-half times longer than wider, so hoops or chandeliers are an excellent choice to create balance. A heart-shaped face has the widest section at the cheekbone and has a narrow forehead, and triangular or heart-shaped earrings flatter this face. Diamond-shaped faces have a narrow chin with a wider forehead and temples, which look terrific in short hoops.

Handbags come in totes, clutches, hoboes, and so many styles! The late Kate Spade designed such whimsical styles, and one of my favorites was the ice cream tote that reminds me of summer! Handbags have become one of the primary ways we express ourselves. Changing your handbag can quickly bring more flair to your sense of style and may help you long for the upcoming seasons such as fall and winter transition to spring and summer. Consider your body shape and size and select a bag that works well with your frame. A large handbag can overwhelm a small or petite body type, yet a medium or large tote may complement a medium or larger body frame.

Shoes can become an obsession for many women. The classic stilettoes with a pointed toe are probably the most flattering type of shoe for all women because they lengthen the leg line and provide balance to your body. You can substitute it with a wedge that is either gold, rose gold, or nude and get pretty much the same effect. Women who have an hourglass figure look incredible in a feminine peep-toe heels because they complement your curves, they are versatile, and they accentuate your defined waist. Chunky sandals can complement someone with thin legs. Some ankle strap shoes only flatter a woman's body if they have long slender legs because they can cut off your height and give the illusion of larger legs. However, if they are worn underneath your pant leg, you do not have the look of enlargement or shorter frame. Platforms also create more height and can provide more comfort if you find stilettoes to be uncomfortable. Dance shoes that have suede in the sole can be wonderful for dancing the night away at the next wedding or formal event! My favorites are ones that have a small platform to provide comfort and height and great balance. English riding boots are very chic with jeans and jodhpurs, and dark colored boots and jeans are incredibly flattering.

Tailor: Tuck, Taper, and Cut

One time when my husband and I visited London, we took a tour of Kensington Palace—the late Princess Diana's home—and I saw a collection of some of her ball gowns. She was a fashion icon, and I discovered that one of the reasons she looked so elegant and her evening wear fit her so well was that the undergarments were sewn into the fabric. The designers must have painstakingly custom designed her attire to glide over her beautiful body! A talented tailor is essential to building your wardrobe. They can help prevent and repair wardrobe malfunctions like sewing undergarments into your actual clothing (i.e., breast cups for backless cocktail attire such as a halter dress). When it comes to purchasing moderate to lower end fashion, a tailor can work magic with the style, and you look like you are wearing couture.

Most reputable tailors are working either in a large retail store or in indoor or outdoor shopping malls. If you are purchasing a somewhat expensive garment at a retail store, it is best to use their tailor because if there is damage done to the clothing, you have some recourse. However, the best tailors are sometimes the ones who have a background in high-end couture experience and have a degree in fashion. Be cognizant of the fact that you can get a quote from the tailor prior to having them do the alterations or buying the merchandise. Therefore, you can make a decision if it is worth the investment.

One of the most flattering tailoring styles is to simply taper a dress, skirt, or alter pants and jeans. This provides a fitted look that high end retail typically offers. Likewise, the hem of your garment has a wow factor (bell bottom pants that kiss the ground) if it is precisely placed where it accentuates your body type. The capri-length pants or jeans may cut you off but work well for girls and women who are tall.

Fabulous and Fit through the Ages

Wardrobe essentials are important to consider as your body changes throughout the seasons and years of your life. Some of the beautiful style icons are over age forty, such as Nicole Kidman who has mastered not only her sense of style, but exudes self-confidence, self-knowledge, and poise. When a woman who feels comfortable in her own skin steps out, all eyes are on them. Self-esteem and self-efficacy are the most important issues that a woman can wear when it comes to fashion. One can have on the most amazing ball gown or designer jeans and feel more beautiful than ever, especially if they have mastered their PQ (positive self-esteem and body esteem) and their FQ (dressing to flatter their figure).

Clearly, during and after pregnancy can be a challenging time for a woman with regard to wardrobe and body image. Actress Jessica Alba is cofounder of The Honest Company, mom to two kids, and serves on the board of Baby2Baby, which is a nonprofit organization that provides supplies for babies. In a candid interview at the gala for Baby2Baby on the red carpet wearing a stunning black lace maternity evening gown and expecting her third baby, she acknowledged that she too struggles with body image during pregnancy. She stated, "I don't feel glamourous at all when I'm pregnant, so it's nice to kind of dress up and feel beautiful." The mom-to-be went on to say, "I usually feel sort of like Humpty Dumpty, slothing around and hormonal, and nothing fits the same. But in this dress, I actually feel kind of pretty."

It is refreshing for celebrities like Alba to share that they too are human and may struggle with their attire and body image issues during pregnancy. Although women look radiant during pregnancy with their glowing complexions and lovely locks, they may not always feel their best. Therefore, it is imperative to find maternity clothes that you feel comfortable and confident wearing. Along the same lines, it is important that we not body shame women who are expecting as most of them are pretty hard on themselves anyway. At a party, I once witnessed a husband bend down and tie his wife's shoes because she was expecting twins and was unable to bend over and as he stood up he kissed her baby bump and said, "You are the most beautiful woman in the world!"

No worries because there is a plethora of fashion tips for these bodily changes. Many years ago, my brother and sister-in-law traveled to India on their trip around the world. The gorgeous colors of fabrics are brilliant, and the pashminas are so luxurious and inexpensive. I was fortunate to receive such a beautiful lavender one as a gift. My niece also gave me a gorgeous silk striped pashmina in all of my favorite colors (lilac, pink, and blue). If you are self-conscious about your arms, but you want to still wear your cocktail dresses, invest in pashminas. You can dress them up or down with a great pair of jeans, and they are functional as well whenever you are traveling. You can wrap up in one on the plane to stay warm or at the theater. You may want to personalize it and monogram it with your initials to make it yours.

In closing, there is no price tag for self-esteem and self-efficacy. It is actually free but takes an investment of time into yourself. Improvement that you make in your fashion quotient will continue to contribute to your overall body esteem quotient. The most expensive couture garments will not work for you if you don't wear them with confidence. Your sense of style impacts your body esteem and is the bow on the beautiful gift package. However, fashion is only one aspect of improving your body esteem quotient, and without self-esteem, there would be no package for the ribbon. Your gift to yourself is to learn to create your signature style that flatters your body and simultaneously builds body esteem.

Chapter 7
Body Shaming and Bullying

"Never be bullied into silence. Never allow yourself to be made a victim. Accept no one's definition of your life; define yourself."
—Harvey Fierstein

Adele is beloved throughout the world for her incredibly raspy voice that is distinct and recognizable. This is not the only thing that is unique about Adele. She's also known to care little about what other people say about her since she has been repeatedly body shamed and long ago stopped looking to others for approval. She talked about body image issues during a Sirius XM Town Hall when she was promoting *25*, and she openly discussed her body image issues just like any other Snapchat-using person on the planet. She stated, "I do have body image problems, for sure, but I don't let them rule my life at all. And there's bigger issues going on in the world than how I might feel about myself and stuff like that." The most profound statement was as follows: "There's only one of you, so why would you want to look like everyone else?"

Dirty Words
Body shaming is defined as the action or practice of humiliating someone by making mocking or critical comments about their body shape or size.

It has become so prevalent due to a certain freedom of opinion shared in social media with people hiding behind their tweets, Facebook, and Instagram remarks. It is directed at others to comment on how they look. But it doesn't only take place online. Body shaming takes place every day on the playground and school bus, in dance or gym class, and at social events and the workplace. Critical comments often mask hostility through joking and even by making passive-aggressive remarks about how much one is eating, how their clothes fit, and on and on and on.

The truth is that we know when someone else is being insensitive, judgmental, or downright cruel. Trust your instincts and intuition! We have felt the sting of the hurtful comments that cut so deep when our face turns red due to embarrassment or when we are so stunned that we do not have a quick comeback. Often those remarks come from a place where they are constantly comparing themselves to others to make sure they "measure up" and have much more to do with them than they have to do with you. But still, the emotional pain can be excruciating, so much so that it may affect your self-esteem and subsequently your desire to go to an event or even a family gathering. Some families can be particularly unkind because their remarks over the years may have made an indelible impact on how we feel about ourselves, particularly in how we look. We can remember with varying amounts of pain every ill-fitting dress or wardrobe malfunction when we were teased and laughed at and yet no one confronted their cruel comments because we chose to feel intimated by them.

Not anymore because times are changing, my friend! I propose that we implement a body esteem etiquette (#BEE) just like we have a business and social etiquette whereby one asserts themselves and no longer tolerates these inappropriate behaviors. Today we have choices in terms of how we would like to be treated and how we allow others to speak to us. My goal in this chapter is to have an open discussion about body bullying and body shaming and how you may have become self-punitive as a result of this. Unlike Adele's assertive reaction to body shaming, you may have been hurt deeply in a way that may still impact how you feel about your body even today. You will learn techniques on how to avoid and cope with body shaming since none of us want to be at war with ourselves about our bodies. They are truly meant to be loved, celebrated, and enjoyed.

Looking to others for validation for your body image or comparing yourself to others inhibits body esteem. If you take to heart the critical remarks others have made, you may become self-deprecating (i.e., If they think I am fat, it must be so!) In other words, if you believe any of the "dirty words" that others have said about your body, you will potentially take over where they left off and body shame yourself. After all, we are hard enough on ourselves, and others body shaming us only makes matters worse. However, you will learn to be assertive and set clear boundaries by denouncing any form of body shaming and not allowing anyone, including a spouse, child, parent, or friend to cross that line and make derogatory remarks about your body, especially if they are veiled as teases or passive aggressive prompts (#BEE).

Furthermore, you are making yourself very vulnerable for feedback about your body if you are making negative comments about yourself in front of others. By doing so, you are participating in setting the environment that says, "It is okay to shame me because I'm doing it myself." This includes pointing out how much weight you've gained or even a general remark about how you don't feel good about your current looks. Often, we offer up these remarks hoping to solicit support or approval to contradict our own feelings, but it often doesn't go that way, and you just end up feeling worse. Of course, I don't want you to sing your own praises if you aren't feeling it. Just as we do with our eating and the four quotients, we really want to build self-efficacy and body esteem, which can take place if we let others know you are off the market for their criticism, comparison, and critique (#BEE)!

Art Therapy

For years we have used art therapy in our clinic to work with body image issues, and it is incredibly therapeutic. Have you ever been body shamed by someone? Pause for a moment and recall the "dirty words" that still may be emblazoned in your memory whether it be you have thunder thighs, a pot belly, or a muffin top! Write these words down and record your feelings at the actual time and how you feel today and examine whether they still affect your body image. You do not have to be an artist, but draw a picture of how you saw yourself after the body shaming and how you see yourself today. Next, draw a picture of how you would like to see your body!

Another art therapy technique is to paint these words on stones and throw them in a lake or sea, symbolic of letting go of those labels. Paint new words on stones that you keep, such as a beautiful smile, physically fit body, and lovely legs and keep these stones and embrace these positive affirmations. Now vow to become assertive and confront anyone who says anything negative about your body. Find your own words such as, "I am not going to allow you to make negative comments about my body or appearance in the future." If this is not honored or respected, then you may choose to distance yourself from or terminate the relationship.

Emma Stone is such a talented actress and someone whose candor and eloquence we routinely appreciate, so it came as no surprise that her response to comments about her weight were so well put. In an interview with *USA Today*, she said, "I firmly believe that nothing really affects you or can really bother you if you don't already feel that way about yourself. I've seen a lot of comments that say, 'Eat a sandwich' or 'She looks sick.' I've been looking at myself in the mirror being mean to myself. I'm not sick. I eat sandwiches. . . . In no way is it my intention to be a bad example. That has been kind of bothering me lately. I've shamed myself for it. We shame each other online. We're always too skinny or too fat or too tall or too short. They're just confirming this feeling I have about myself. I'm trying to figure my body out. It bothers me because I care so much about young girls. We're shaming each other and we're shaming ourselves and it sucks."

Body Bullying

I think we can all take some valuable lessons from Emma Stone's playbook and one in particular is to not buy into how others see you so you can prevent body bullying. Bullying may be defined as the use of force, threat, or coercion to abuse, intimidate, or aggressively dominate others. The aggressive behavior is often times repetitive and habitual, which breeds more anxiety and fear for the victim. One fundamental prerequisite is the perception, by the bully or by others, of an imbalance of social or physical power, which distinguishes bullying from conflict.

Maladaptive behaviors that assert such domination can be manifested in the form of verbal harassment or threat, physical assault, or coercion, and can be directed repeatedly towards particular targets. Studies show that the bully often rationalizes his or her behavior based on differences in social class, race, religion, gender, sexual orientation, appearance, behavior, body language, personality, reputation, lineage, strength, size, or ability.

My husband and I got engaged at the Raffles Hotel in the Long Bar in Singapore, and he loves to say he had too many Singapore Slings, their famous cocktail! The truth is, he proposed before the cocktails arrived! We later were escorted back to our hotel in a rickshaw in the pouring rain! That was the best ride of my life, and I will never forget it! The wonderful experience of having been engaged in such a lovely place also holds fond memories of the melting pot of different cultures for both of us.

If we are going to cease body shaming and body bullying, it is essential to embrace our differences. Exposing yourself without judgement to a myriad of cultures and ethnic and religious backgrounds makes life more interesting. I have had the privilege to work with people from all over the world (i.e., South Africa, South America, Asia, Europe), which has not only broadened my horizons, but actually made my life much richer and fuller.

My support system is diverse: my dear German friend who provides thought-provoking conversations about music, art and literature; my Catholic friend who has inspired me by her example to overcome obstacles; my friend who is a late bloomer like myself; my friends and relatives who are independent thinkers who encourages me to see all sides of an argument; my lovely niece and her beautiful wife; my Jewish friends who provide belly laughs; my gorgeous friend who was a former Miss Texas and is beautiful on the inside and out; and my Greek friend who is incredibly kindhearted. In lieu of excluding others who may be different or unique, I think we must be more inclusive to overcome body bullying and embrace cultural differences.

Methods of coercion such as intimidation are often used by the bully, and for this reason alone it is vitally important to not allow others to exercise power and control over you. It is important to remember that one can only be controlled or intimated by others if you allow yourself to be. Feeling powerless over a situation—or yourself, for that matter—robs one of self-esteem and body esteem. Research shows that bullying must meet the following criteria: hostile intent, imbalance of power, and repetition over a period of time. Therefore, bullying may be defined as the activity of repeated, aggressive behavior intended to hurt another individual, physically, mentally, or emotionally.

Take a moment to examine if the following synonyms (i.e., dirty words) that are associated with bullying have impacted you. Write a letter in first person to the bully that you may or may not choose to send describing how this has affected or is currently affecting you and your body image psychologically. Next, write a letter to yourself with words of encouragement and empowerment and be explicit about how you will no longer be a victim.

Dirty Words:
Mock

Humiliate

Embarrass

Taunt

Berate

Abuse

Ridicule

Defame

Words of Encouragement and Empowerment:
Hope

Autonomy

Respect

Boundaries

Self-respect

Self-esteem

Unique

Positive Body Talk

My Body, Not Yours

Types of Bullying

Bullying is divided into four basic types of abuse: emotional, verbal, physical, and cyber. There are many types of bullying, and although we are focusing on body bullying, it seems relevant to have an understanding of other types of bullying that may have had psychological repercussions on one's body image. For this reason, it is imperative to be able to recognize other types of bullying for prevention since I have worked with patients who have experienced workplace bullying and gay bullying, and the residual effect was the development of an eating disorder or poor body image.

Physical

The "Me Too" and "Time's Up" movements have certainly brought to light the significance of standing up for yourself and confronting any perpetrator. As a society we are moving in the direction of having a "no tolerance" policy for body shaming and body bullying. I applaud the courage and strength it takes to overcome any traumatic event. I have great respect and admiration for my patients who have had the courage to seek my help and overcome these issues. You are truly my heroes, and it has been an honor and privilege to share your journey from overcoming the role of a victim to watching you acquire emotional strength, endurance, and empowerment! I applaud you!

This type of bullying aims to physically hurt someone's body or damages their possessions. Physically bullying is rarely the first form of bullying that the victim will experience as it seems to escalate from verbal bullying to potential physical violence. This often seems to manifest with sexual abuse, date rape, sexual misconduct, or sexual harassment. Equip yourself with healthy habits such as avoiding intoxication or taking drugs and be aware of any circumstance where you might be slipped drugs. Establish a safety plan where you can contact someone if necessary. Trust your instincts and judgement at the first signs of inappropriate behavior and do not be afraid to speak up or seek help. No means no, not maybe!

Verbal

Verbal bullying is one of the most common types of bullying. It typically involves mostly girls and women due to the more negative emotional devastation. A classic example is a boss who attempts to bully someone who reports to him in an attempt to dominate and control with their superiority and power.

Many fear being the "whistle blower" if they report this to human resources and worry about the consequences of not finding another job if they are terminated or choose to resign. This may manifest itself with the victim losing or gaining weight due to the extreme levels of stress and the power and control dynamic. Please be cognizant of the fact that others may be experiencing verbal bullying, and you have the right to protect yourself and prevent others from suffering.

Relational

This type of bullying is done with the intent to damage someone's reputation or place in a hierarchy or social standing, and it can also be linked to physical and verbal bullying. Relational bullying is more common among youth and particularly girls (i.e., bullying the new girl at school because others are threatened or jealous of her beauty), and it may persist for a long time since it is not overt.

This seems more prevalent among girls who are ostracized because they may be considered the "good girls" who do not use drugs or alcohol, never act out, and are not sexually active. These girls are often rejected by their peers because they do not conform to the aforementioned behaviors. These children and adolescents seem to be the ones that are more at risk for eating disorders or poor body image. Over time social isolation sets in, and they become incredibly lonely. It is important to remember that, generally speaking, the good girls have a high moral standard, but the rejection from their peers often creates feelings of inadequacy, anxiety, stress, and depression.

Cyberbullying

Chrissy Teigen is a Twitter phenomenon, author of the cookbook *Cravings* (which I absolutely love), and multitalented model who has often been the subject of judgmental remarks. She was body shamed at the 2018 Emmy Awards, with trolls talking about her post pregnancy weight from son Miles. She responded to the trolls in her typical hilarious style by showing them she simply does not have time to be shamed for her body. Let's give new mothers a break! Let every mother celebrate her beautiful baby without the instant worry of how their body has changed.

Cyberbullying is any bullying done through the use of technology to harass, threaten, embarrass, or target another person. It is important to teach our children and adolescents to be cognizant of cyberbullying, and watchdog organizations have been designed to contain the spread of cyberbullying. When an adult is involved, it is referred to as cyber-harassment or cyberstalking, a crime that can have legal consequences and involves jail time.

This includes email, instant messaging, social networking sites, text messages, and cell phones. The psychological ramifications of cyberbullying are devastating to one's body image, and it is imperative to exercise good judgement before you post or give someone else information that is considered confidential. Have a conversation with your children and adolescents and discuss the negative consequences of cyberbullying and methods of prevention to protect them.

Characteristics of the Bully and Accomplices

Imagine what a bully looks like behind his/her mask of wanting to taunt or terrorize you. Take a snapshot of the bully in your mind's eye and reframe the way you see them. A bully can psychologically project his insecurities and vulnerabilities onto his victims. Studies have shown that envy and resentment are the motives, and there is a mixed bag in terms of their self-esteem; some are arrogant and narcissistic, and some may use their bullying as a tool to conceal their shame or anxiety or boost their self-esteem by demeaning others.

The most interesting research from psychologist Roy Baumeister asserts that people who are prone to abusive behavior tend to have inflated but fragile egos. Bullying may also result from a genetic predisposition or a brain abnormality in the bully. Many have risk factors such as depression, personality disorders, obsessive compulsive tendencies, poor impulse control in regard to anger and use of force, addiction to aggressive behaviors, and a strong need to dominate and control others. However, this does not give a bully—or anyone, for that matter—the right to dominate and attempt to control you!

Overcome Victimization

Victims of bullying often have characteristics that make them more vulnerable to being bullied such as being physically weak, easily emotionally distraught, perceived as overweight, or a physical deformity. However, I have seen numerous cases where the victim is passive and conflict avoidant.

Strengthen your skills and empower yourself to overcome issues that make you more vulnerable. Learn new social skills, become more assertive, and implement conflict resolution skills. We have taught the aforementioned life skills in our clinic, and they work beautifully. There are many workbooks online that can teach you these skills. It is important to remember that in order to overcome the victim role, you must begin to see yourself in a different light. If you reframe your body image and do not allow others to victimize you as you gain more self-esteem and self-confidence, you can no longer be a victim to anyone. You be you!

Parenting and Bullying

My clinical impressions are that most parents want to be loving and nurturing and utilize healthy parenting techniques. However, studies show that parents who may displace their anger, hostility, insecurities, or have a persistent need to dominate and control their children in extreme ways have been proven to increase the likelihood that their own children will in turn become overly aggressive and controlling toward their peers. The American Psychological Association advises that parents who suspect their children may be engaging in bullying should carefully consider the examples they may be setting for their children. Observe your own behavior and instead of feeling guilty or frustrated, learn new parenting skills or become more psychologically sophisticated and manage your stress in ways that do not spill over to your children.

Conversely, if you are parenting your child or adolescent who is non-assertive, an approval seeker, and conflict avoidant, you may want to teach them more social skills since these personality traits may set them up to be vulnerable to bullies. Teaching them to have autonomy, to not be afraid to seek help or guidance, and to overcome their fear of rejection will serve them well in the future as a means of prevention from bullying. Similarly, teaching your children and adolescents body esteem etiquette (#BEE) and the consequences of bullying is paramount.

A New Vista

I love looking at my husband's photography, as this is the way he expresses his creative temperament. He often describes how he views the subject matter in a positive manner while he is engaged in street photography (i.e., children playing sports in the Philippines or families laughing and playing with their toddlers on the beach). While he is paragliding, he takes pictures and later turns them into magnificent videos with music we select together. He spends hours perfecting the photos and capturing the desired effect with his landscape and portrait photography. I marvel at his talent and how he seems to find value and beauty in his surroundings. I consider all of his photography a treasure trove that we will have forever to reflect on our travels and experiences.

I know it is possible to consistently find beauty within ourselves and in others (#BEE). I am not suggesting that you should not invest in changes that you want to make, but I do recommend that you take action on what you want to modify. For example, body shaming exists on reality TV and sitcoms that use actors or actresses who are too underweight or overweight as the basis of many of the show's jokes. This is no joking matter because watching this perpetuates body shaming and body bullying.

In addition, it has become more commonplace to criticize aspects of our bodies as some type of bonding experience with our friends; it somehow makes us feel connected and united. Somehow it became endearing and funny to be self-deprecating. But even when joking around, there is both truth and shame in every self-critical remark you make. Even more damaging is participating in making derogatory comments about others when they are not present.

Change the Conversation

Selena Gomez grew up in the spotlight and has subsequently suffered years of body shaming from fans and haters alike. In 2015, the singer and actress shared that she sought therapy after being body shamed publicly. More recently, she clapped back at fans who commented on a photo of her wearing a bikini on Instagram. More celebrities like Selena are not holding back but confronting this verbal abuse and changing the conversation. I challenge you to make a concerted effort to no longer make negative comments about anyone's looks, from yourself to celebrities to supermodels and begin to notice how many times you are tempted to comment on yourself or others.

These remarks and the thoughts that precede them have crept into our daily lives to such an extent that often we are not cognizant of the fact that we are doing this. This type of body shaming (criticizing yourself or others because of some aspect of physical appearance) can lead to a vicious cycle of judgement and hurt feelings. Make a commitment to yourself that you will not engage in this conversation and change the subject by saying "Ladies, let's please talk about something more fun and interesting!"

I have been amazed to see how often women will plan a fun day with friends at a spa or a nail salon and then spend the entire time talking about what they hate about their bodies and what they want to change. Where is the value in that? The next time you experience the "shame binge," try gently telling others that you've made a commitment to only appreciate your body and the bodies of others and immediately point out a few things for each woman present that you appreciate about their looks, and more importantly, their spirit and being as a whole.

In general, some of the messages from the media and from each other often imply that we should want to change, that we must care about looking slimmer or smaller. And if we don't, we worry that we are at risk of being the target of someone else's body shaming comments. What people say about you behind your back is really none of your business because it simply does not matter what others think when it comes to your body image. It only matters how you see yourself!

If you have been engaged in body shaming for so long that you don't even recognize it, here are some of the telltale signs that you may want to consider for shaming yourself and others:

1. Having critical thoughts about your body that are judgmental or doing a comparative analysis with your own body and someone else. ("She is so much thinner than me and I hate my thighs.")
2. Criticizing another person's body in their presence or behind their back. ("OMG-I can't believe she is wearing that with her fat belly.")
3. Making derogatory remarks about one's appearance to their face or behind their back in a passive-aggressive style when you are angry or upset. ("That outfit does not flatter your figure and it makes your butt look even bigger.")
4. Group shaming where you point fingers and selectively target someone and poke fun at their body. ("She is the biggest girl in our club.")
5. Secretively shaming yourself or others mentally with obsessive compulsive thoughts about your body. ("How am I ever going to fit into my wedding gown if I keep eating?")
6. Projecting your impressions onto others regarding poor body image. ("I hope she doesn't wear horizontal stripes today because they make her look so heavy.")

Instead:

1. Distance yourself from others who body shame you or obsess about body image issues.
2. Be bold and assert yourselves when others are body shaming because you can make a dramatic difference.
3. Attempt to be the one who sets an example about body positivity.
4. Acknowledge positive mental statements about your body and others.
5. If you are concerned about a friend or loved one who seems to have an eating disorder or body image issues, express your compassion and encourage them to seek help.
6. Reach out to others who may have been body shamed or bullied and show them empathy by not excluding them from social events.

Body Esteem Movement (#BEM)

I challenge you to implement my philosophy that I have developed over the years of working with body image issues, called Body Esteem Movement (#BEM). Body shaming and body bullying often lead to feelings of inadequacy and perpetuate the concept that we should judge ourselves and those around us based on body type and perceived figure flaws. However, I believe the #BEM can gain momentum and revolutionize not only the way we see our own bodies, but also to no longer criticize other bodies. This is a golden opportunity for us to come together and appreciate not only our similarities, but our differences in our glorious bodies. There are endless possibilities when it comes to #BEM:

- No longer tolerate body shaming and body bullying.
- Connect with others who want to engage in the #BEM for emotional support.
- Change our description and language to a more positive tone when speaking about our body and others (#BEE).
- Show kindness and compassion to others who may be different than you.
- Understand the concepts of body bullying and prevent yourself from becoming a victim or overcome your victimization.

Prevention and Wellness

If you really want to make a difference and support #BEM, you may want to invest in bullying prevention, which is a collective effort to prevent, reduce, and cease bullying. Many campaigns for bullying prevention are designated throughout the world: Anti-Bullying Day; Anti-Bullying Week, International Day of Pink, and International STAND UP to Bullying Day. The National Bullying Prevention Month combats body bullying such as weight shaming in school systems, which has reached an epidemic proportion in today's modern society. Anti-bullying laws in the United States have been enacted in twenty-three of its fifty states, making bullying in schools illegal.

Body bullying and body shaming have a significant psychological effect on one's emotional and physical well-being. If that individual already experiences low self-esteem and poor body image, it may make matters worse and can develop into a formal eating disorder. Therefore, it is essential to promote body positivity not only in the classroom, but in extracurricular activities such as sports like swimming and volleyball. It is essential that teachers and leaders of these extracurricular activities act as role models and provide a safe environment for the students.

In order to prevent or counteract bullying, you must not ignore it because it often escalates, and the other choices are to confront the bully or seek help from an authority figure such as parents, school counselors, human resources, and so on. As a bystander you can play an important role in responding to bullying, as doing nothing encourages it to continue while taking action, even small steps, will improve the situation.

There are many ways that one can preserve and promote #BEM and stamp out body shaming and bullying. Make a concerted effort to complement others on aspects such as personality traits like determination. Emphasize other strengths like academic performance and minimize making one's appearance or body shape be so prominent. Draw a line in the sand by setting healthy boundaries where you do not talk about your body shame and encourage others to do the same. Do not let comments go when someone body shames you. Assert yourself and let them know this is not acceptable behavior.

In my experience, many bullies are cowards, and once confronted by an individual or a group this often disarms them from continuing to bully others. Setting healthy boundaries promotes #BEM and allows you to be a role model for protecting yourself and others against body shaming. Whether it be at a luncheon, the classroom, with family members, or at the office, your positivity will provide an environment that is conducive for body esteem. Lastly, two heads are better than one so collaborate, communicate, and support others on how to handle these matters.

Therefore, building strong support systems where others are educated on prevention of bullying and not hiding out of fear can help us all avoid being bullied. It is important to remember that eating disorders are complex illnesses, and while bullying does not necessarily cause eating disorders, it could play a role in the development of one. In closing, it is vitally important to remember that there is strength in numbers, and we all have a responsibility to ban body bullying in our environment so we can create a life-affirming environment where we feel safe and secure.

Chapter 8
Baby Your Body

"The human body is the best work of art."
—Jess C. Scott

*D*o you recall the scent of a freshly bathed baby with all of the smells of baby powder and soap? The aromas are so fresh and clean, and the baby's skin is so silky smooth! Parents take such care of their babies to welcome them into the world and protect them. Learning to baby your own body is crucial to body esteem. Yes, baby yourself! This concept is often misunderstood, and many believe that if you are focused on yourself that you may become too self-absorbed. Maintaining your psychological and physical health allows you to take care of yourself and your loved ones. In addition, you can assume the many roles that you play in your life whether you are a husband, wife, daughter, son, parent, or single.

Kate Winslet said, "As a child, I never heard one woman say to me, 'I love my body.' Not my mother, my elder sister, my best friend. No one woman has ever said, 'I am so proud of my body.' So, I make sure to say it to Mia [her daughter], because a positive physical outlook has to start at an early age." Parents are often the most influential role model in their children's lives, and you can teach your kids to have healthy body image.

My clinical impressions are that parents want to be supportive when it comes to positive body talk and are open to parenting techniques that address this issue.

As I was writing this book, many friends and colleagues inquired about how to cope with body image issues with their children and adolescents. It inspired me to write another book for preteens and teens after completing this one because introducing them to body esteem at a young age is essential. It coincides with my philosophy that "Healthy beginnings have happy endings!" I believe that parents can be proactive by using preventive techniques to educate their children on body esteem. Do not wait until an issue arises like someone body shames your child, but educate them on techniques of the four quotients to equip them with coping mechanisms. I think this is equally as important as teaching good manners, drug prevention, sex education, and other life skills.

Positive Body Talk for Parents and Kids

One of the most effective ways to foster body esteem is to make sure you as a parent have a healthy relationship with food and are vigilant so that the impact of your attitudes and behaviors with regard to your body is a positive one. Whether you are a parent, grandparent, aunt or uncle, single, or have no children, the following are healthy techniques that instill body esteem:

- Avoid making derogatory comments about your body and others, and use positive language when describing your food intake such as "flavorful" and "delectable."
- If negative body talk comes up in a conversation or via media pause and take this opportunity to educate your children, yourself, or others on how this is inappropriate.
- Avoid fad diets and obsessing about food or body topics.
- Emphasize the significance of psychological and physical health as a form of wellness and prevention.
- Learn to have an appreciation for other aspects of yourself such as personality traits, skills, talents, academic performance, and career development.

- Listen and process your children's or loved ones concerns about their body and encourage them to speak openly about this issue.
- Make teasing off limits with regard to weight, body shape, or looks.
- Turn off all electronics during meal time and limit exposure to social media.
- Do not be a helicopter parent where you hover over your children or loved ones and micromanage their food and exercise routine.
- Avoid being a lawnmower parent where you overprotect your child; instead, allow them to experience valuable life lessons such as negotiating conflict with others or how to handle failure.

Family Affair and Body Esteem

The average adolescent spends approximately nine hours per day using media for their enjoyment and pleasure according to a report by Common Sense Media. Unfortunately, they may only spend less than an average of ten minutes a day talking to their parents. During the social media time a teenager may be bombarded with thousands of messages about the "ideal body." Research shows that these unrealistic and unattainable portrayals of beauty can wreak havoc on their body image. Set limits for your children and adolescents and yourself because it is important to have a balance, and by not spending excessive time on technology one builds social skills, interpersonal relationships, and communication techniques. The following are methods on how to combat harmful effects of media not only for yourself, but for your family as well:

- Become media literate and understand that the concepts one is exposed to via smartphones and other electronic devices may be an idealized version of beauty.
- Have candid conversations about body image and teach concepts on how to build body esteem.
- Maximize the opportunity to have discussions about unhealthy body image when it presents itself like looking through a magazine or watching a movie.

- Emphasize the importance of prevention by making time for yourself and your family to exercise, eat balanced meals, manage stress, and maintain physical exams for heart health, brain health, and wellness.
- Designate a certain amount of time that kids can have access to technology like social media, and maximize the moment by turning off electronics like during carpool.
- Have a family meeting where you have a climate that is conducive for open communication where you discuss issues and the highs and lows of each day.

Beauty Is in the Eye of the Beholder

Some of the people who I have found most attractive tend to have unique characteristics like my husband's gap in his front teeth, which is incredibly sexy! I love seeing crow's feet from smiling, and adorable freckles or scars. The time is now since one of the health trends for 2018 was to embrace the body positive movement. This actually originates with each and every one of us making a concerted effort to be a part of this movement. The Positive Body Movement encourages people to adopt more forgiving and affirming attitudes towards their bodies, with the goal of improving overall health and well-being. This movement was designed to help people not be at war with their bodies and learn to lead a more balanced lifestyle.

Moreover, the grass roots of the movement was to inspire others to value their health and unique beauty. Beauty is in the eye of the beholder! It is fascinating that in their teens Connie Sobczak and Elizabeth Scott created the body positive campaign in 1996 in their living room along with some friends. Clearly, they were wise beyond their years because their mission statement was to accept unique and realistic body images that lead to a more balanced self-loving life. Although it was initially developed based on body politics and social stigmas, it later included size discrimination based on height and weight. In essence, the body positivity movement is dramatically changing how we view our bodies and how we are transitioning from nonacceptance and among our bodies.

Piece of Cake and Peace of Mind: Celebrate Body Esteem

Over the years when I have hosted a charity event that I am chairing, I like to serve champagne and cupcakes because everyone seems to love them both! A British saying is "cheap and cheerful," and the cupcakes and cheap champagne fit the bill! I challenge you to have a party for one or for your family and friends, and make a commitment to build body esteem. My wish for you is to experience peace of mind as you enjoy your piece of cake! Here are some ideas that you may want to consider:

- A cupcake party where you implement positive body talk and no longer say anything derogatory about your body or others.
- A sheet cake party where you commit to "no more chronic dieting and emotional eating" and incorporate normalized eating by using the hunger rating scale and list on "What's Normal."
- A two-tiered cake where you jumpstart a healthy lifestyle by implementing techniques that promote psychological and physical health.
- A three-tiered cake where you celebrate your body and all of your strengths such as personality traits, intellectual capabilities, brain health, and specific body parts (i.e., breasts or legs).
- A designer Chanel cake where you curate your own closet (#CYOC), become your own stylist (#BYOS), and flaunt your favorite features (#FYFF) that flatter your beautiful body!
- A petit fours where you set goals to implement the four quotients that comprise body esteem quotient (BEQ).
- An ice cream cake where you make a commitment to implement all of the food groups and an exercise prescription.

Everyone should design their own wellness program that addresses their needs and preferences for improving body esteem quotient (BEQ). The best method to use in creating your wellness profile is to implement each one of the following quotients: psychological quotient (PQ), nutrition quotient (NQ), exercise quotient (EQ), and fashion quotient (FQ). These components may vary depending on your physical and psychological needs, and the following quotients may inspire you to have a better quality of life.

PQ | Psychology Quotient

- Take time for yourself one hour per day to recharge your batteries via listening to music, playing scrabble, or taking a cat nap!

- Turn off all electronics during meal time, when it is socially unacceptable, and two hours prior to bedtime.

- Make time to do something you find pleasurable and relaxing such as going to the art museum, a musical or concert, a sporting event like a tennis or golf tournament, or attending a charity event.

- Complete a comprehensive psychological test battery with a mental health professional and improve your mental health.

- Adopt or rescue an animal that provides unconditional love or sign up for English or Western horseback riding lessons to counteract loneliness.

- Complete a family genogram to improve your family of origin functioning or learn conflict resolutions skills to improve interpersonal relationships.

- Seek out professional counseling or biofeedback to help you manage your stress and improve your psychological functioning.

- Join a support group where others share similar issues such as divorce recovery, eating disorders, or smoking cessation.

- Go online to a reputable website like Psychology Today and complete assessments for stress, anxiety, depression, emotional eating, quality of life assessment, and personality inventories.

- Schedule a mother/daughter or husband/wife or one just for you at a weekend retreat or spa.

NQ | Nutrition Quotient

- Schedule a consult with a licensed dietitian and complete a nutritional analysis and vitamin supplement assessment to make sure you are getting the antioxidants and nutritional needs for your body.

- Provide yourself with a snack before bedtime like hot herbal tea and Godiva dark chocolate to avoid deprivation.

- Tickle your taste buds by cooking recipes from other cultures like Germany or the Caribbean, and share facts about the country for a wonderful culinary experience.

- Add veggies into one pot meals to ensure you are meeting the requirement for fruits and vegetables (i.e., add celery, carrots, and onion to your spaghetti sauce or kale or baby spinach on your favorite sandwich or soup).

- Start a dinner club or progressive dinner party to celebrate with food and connect with others.

- Hire a chef or sign up for cooking classes.

- Dine like you are in Paris and select several appetizers in lieu of an entree or split a larger entrée and dessert since this often pleases one's palette due to the variety.

- Keep healthy snacks at all times in your purse and desk and plan meals ahead of time such as the weekend for weekday dinners.

- Hydrate your body with eight to ten glasses of water per day and limit alcoholic beverages that can dehydrate you.

- Busy people tend to use food as a reward for their behavior and make sure you are not depriving yourself of the foods you love, but also using other positive reinforces like downloading on your playlist.

- Assemble some meals in lieu of cooking to save time (i.e., my recipe in my upcoming cookbook with a rotisserie chicken makes a delectable cranberry chicken salad or caprese salad with heirloom tomatoes and basil pesto).

- Pack your lunch each day and make sure you are eating a variety to conserve costs (i.e., recipes from my upcoming cookbook: corn chowder, roasted vegetable panini, leftover manicotti or eggplant parmesan, grilled chicken, shrimp, and beef satay with peanut sauce, or Southwestern Caesar salad).

- Teach your children to grocery shop and cook or assemble ten meals before they leave home so they can began to have a healthy relationship with food and nourish their bodies.

EQ | Exercise Quotient

- Sign up for ice skating or ice dancing lessons by yourself or with a partner.

- Schedule seasonal goals to travel to various places to participate or compete in your sport or dance competitions to keep you motivated.

- Work out at home on a stationary bike or peloton to save time in lieu going to the gym, or purchase a desk that provides exercise while you work.

- Multi-task your exercise program as you simultaneously engage your cognitive abilities (i.e., learn a new language such as Italian) to improve your brain health and physical health.

- Schedule four workouts per week in lieu of five and on one day incorporate fartlek intervals (steady activity with increased speed or elevation).

- Schedule a workout like a bike ride or rollerblading with a friend or book a personal trainer, which insures dependability and commitment.

- Take swimming lessons or join a Master's swim club.

- Plan to participate in a biathlon or triathlon and train in advance.

- Sign up for a race for a cause like the American Heart Association.

- Sign up for a dance class like ballet, hip hop, salsa, ballroom dancing, modern, or jazz.

- Go rock climbing or hiking with a group of friends or by yourself.

- Take up yoga or Pilates either individually or in a group class.

- Join a dinner and dance club and meet new friends who share your same passion for dancing.

FQ | Fashion Quotient

- Seek out an app for the latest trends in fashion before purchasing any garments and carefully assess if it coincides with your preferences for fashion.

- Purchase clothes at a designer consignment store because they are gently worn and more economical.

- Purchase a fashionable wardrobe that you feel confident wearing for your workouts.

- As you achieve your fitness and nutrition goals, purchase a new outfit each season that flatters your figure.

- Find the collection of designers and styles that work best for you and order online in lieu of going to the shopping malls or boutiques to save time.

- Hire someone to redesign and reorganize your closet in a systematic manner where it is more efficient to reach for outfits that you have cataloged.

- Purchase purse inserts so you do not have to completely change out your handbag and buy articles of clothing that go from day until night with a quick change of accessories (i.e., chandelier or tassel earrings).

- Place your purses and shoes in clear containers to protect them from dust and you have a better visual while styling your wardrobe.

- Change over your wardrobe and closet each season so you can create excitement and anticipate the upcoming season.

- Do a makeover or attend a fashion show and luncheon to learn more about what enhances your natural beauty and become more fashion forward.

- Strategically build one aspect of your wardrobe such as accessories and attend an event or trunk show in a retail store to learn about scarf tying or how to accessorize your clothing.

- Hire a personal shopper or stylist to educate yourself on becoming more fashion forward if you do not feel comfortable styling your wardrobe.

- Build a personal relationship with a salesperson at a retail store or boutique who understands your sense of style and can partner with you to help build your wardrobe and contacts you when there is a sale.

Daydreams

Don't quit your daydreams! Susan Boyle is a Scottish singer who received international attention when she was a contestant on *Britain's Got Talent* in 2009. Unfortunately, she was laughed at by the audience and eyes were rolled when she announced that she wanted to become a famous singer like Elaine Paige. When she opened her mouth and began to sing "I Dreamed a Dream" from *Les Misérables*, the audience and judges were stunned by her angelic voice. As I watched the YouTube video, tears were streaming down my face when I heard her lovely voice. She went on to release her first album entitled *I Dreamed a Dream*, which became the United Kingdom's best-selling debut album of all time. Her second album, which was called *The Gift*, became only the third act ever to top both the UK and US album charts twice in the same year. She has subsequently released four more albums that have been equally successful.

She later returned to the stage at *Britain's Got Talent* as a guest and sang "You'll See." She also performed a duet with Elaine Page singing "I Know Him So Well." Today she holds the record for the fastest selling female debut album of all time. In her book entitled *Dreams Can Come True* she explores her amazing story of rags-to-riches. She recently released a new CD called *What a Wonderful World*.

What most people do not know about Susan Boyle is that she suffers from Asperger syndrome, which is a neurodevelopmental disorder that manifests itself with difficulties with social skills and communication. As a child, she was bullied and ostracized by others, and stones were actually thrown at her. Many adults who suffer from this disorder develop anxiety and depression. Once she was told about her condition, she said, "I feel relieved." She recently was diagnosed with type 2 diabetes, and her doctors told her she needed to lose weight for her health, so she lost twenty-eight pounds. Despite many cruel remarks along the way made about her body and appearance and a history of being ridiculed and bullied, she prevailed.

Now, nearly a decade later, she returned to the spotlight to once again perform for *America's Got Talent: The Champions*. In an interview she said, "*Britain's Got Talent* absolutely changed my life," she continued, "People saw me as somebody quite ordinary. I lived alone with my cat, Pebbles. Now I've sold twenty million records! Wow, even I'm overwhelmed. This has helped me fulfill the dream I've had since I was five."

Susan has spent a great deal of her earnings on philanthropic endeavors and has become a role model for so many people with dreams, which is why she felt the timing was right to return to *Champions*. "I think I'm a champion for maybe those who don't have the confidence to do things, for those who don't have a voice and for those who people tend to ignore," she shared. "I feel I'm a champion for them." Showing her virtuoso vocal range and musical mastery, Boyle wowed the audience with a heartwarming, beautiful rendition of the Rolling Stones' "Wild Horses," and it was flawless!

The Spice Girls star Mel B sent the crowd into a frenzy of excitement as she stood up and pressed the Golden Buzzer for the songstress, sending Susan Boyle into the finals for *America's Got Talent: The Champions*. As gold confetti showered Susan and the crowd, she was asked how she felt about getting the Golden Buzzer. She said all choked up and sweetly, "I'm happy and very humbled. Thank you so much." Susan Boyle exemplifies two values that I try to live by and those are to "never judge a book by its cover" and "dreams really do come true."

Body Esteem Movement (#BEM): Be Your Own Kind of Beautiful

My dream is to create the Body Esteem Movement (#BEM) by embracing "Be Your Own Kind of Beautiful." I dream that accepting that we each have different, equally extraordinary bodies becomes a way of life. I dream of the day where we change the conversation to positive body talk. Being a victim of sexual misconduct or sexual harassment should no longer be tolerated in our society. I dream of a time that body shaming and body bullying will no longer exist. I dream of maintaining mental and physical well-being through preventive healthcare and wellness. I dream that in our near future we no longer impose societal norms or a paradigm of an unrealistic standard of beauty upon ourselves or others. I believe in you! And I dream of the day where you began to believe in yourself! My ultimate dream is that I will inspire others to achieve body esteem and experience "piece of cake and peace of mind!" And I believe that you can help these dreams come true!

Reference List

Introduction

psychologydictionary.org/body-esteem/

Read, Herbert. *The Meaning of Art*, page 127. Faber, 1931.

foxnews.com/health/
    stretching-beauty-ballerina-misty-copeland-on-her-body-struggles

Friedman, Vanessa. "A New Age in French-Modeling," *New York Times*,
    May 2017.

huffingtonpost.com/scarlett-johansson/the-skinny_b_186233.html

Chapter 1

womanmagazine.co.uk/oman-magazine/william-kate-royal-love-story-65016

huffingtonpost.com/entry/aretha-franklin-liz-smith-new-york-post-
    letter_us_5b75a015e4b02b415d76a5a3

time.com/4400847/serena-williams-quotes/

glamour.com/story/serena-williamss-played-for-the-moms-speech-at-
    wimbledon-had-royals-near-tears

web.stanford.edu/~kcarmel/CC_BehavChange_Course/readings/
    Bandura_Selfefficacy_1994.htm

instyle.com/beauty/makeup/jennifer-lopez-inglot-beauty-routine

stress.org/self-assessment/

webmd.com/diet/features/stress-weight-gain#1

forbes.com/sites/forbesagencycouncil/2018/03/30/
    all-you-need-to-know-to-motivate-millennials/#6400fc8260ae

cbsnews.com/news/8-tips-for-losing-weight-after-pregnancy-21-11-2008/
eonline.com/Rosie Huntington Hunt on losing weight on ENews on
    episode
bodylogicmd.com/for-women/hormones-and-weight-gain
psychologytoday.com/us/blog/the-path-passionate-happiness/201611/
    how-remain-optimistic-through-change

Chapter 2

greatist.com/grow/100-years-womens-body-image
foodtimeline.org/foodsandwiches.html
sbs.com.au/news/why-do-women-cry-more-than-men
Burgess, Lana. "Eight Benefits of Crying." medicalnewstoday.com/
    articles/319631.php
Galen, Nicole. "How Do I Stop Stress Eating?" medicalnewstoday.com/
    articles/320935.php
Batts Allen, Ashley and Mark R. Leary. "Self-Compassion, Stress, and
    Coping." ncbi.nlm.nih.gov/pmc/articles/PMC2914331/
psychologytoday.com/us/blog/diet-is-4-letter-word/201304/
    healing-emotional-eating
eatingdisorders.org.au/eating-disorders/disordered-eating-a-dieting
countryliving.com/life/entertainment/a20703527/
    kelly-clarkson-weight-gain-body-image/
livestrong.com/article/209554-jealousy-in-women/
universityofcalifornia.edu/
    Study+at+University+of+California,+Berkeley+shows+that+as+
    social+media+evolves,+the+popularity+of+photo
cbsnews.com/news/too-many-selfies-you-may-have-selfitis/
bluezones.com/2012/07/are-you-heart-hungry/
waldeneatingdisorders.com/what-we-treat/binge-eating-disorder/
    potential-causes-of-and-risk-factors-for-binge-eating-disorder/
health.harvard.edu/mind-and-mood/a-guide-to-cognitive-fitness
edcatalogue.com/dsm-5-eating-disorders/
health.harvard.edu/heart-health/tuning-in-how-music-may-affect-your-heart
cooperaerobics.com/Health-Tips/Stress-Less/Laughing-Away-Stress.aspx

mnn.com/family/pets/
    stories/11-studies-that-prove-pets-are-good-your-health
independent.co.uk/life-style/health-and-families/nature-body-image-
    positive-countryside-study-anglia-ruskin-perdana-university-
    college-london-a8172651.html

Chapter 3

vogue.com/article/
    ashley-graham-2016-plus-size-supermodel-fashion-disrupter
independent.co.uk/life-style/i-weigh-jameela-jamil-instagram-kristen-
    bell-emmy-rossum-weight-movement-a8489371.html
today.ucf.edu/too-fat-to-be-a-princess-study-shows-young-girls-worry-
    about-body-image/
thisisinsider.com/does-gigi-hadid-have-hashimotos-disease-what-
    is-it-2016-12
usatoday.com/story/news/nation-now/2018/02/01/singles-america-
    match-survey-dating-what-makes-good-sex-bad-sex/1078507001/
goredforwomen.org/fight-heart-disease-
    women-go-red-women-official-site/
    about-go-red/
apa.org/news/press/releases/2017/08/fat-shaming.aspx
psychologyofeating.com/chronic-dieting/Chapter 4
coach.nine.com.au/2017/06/01/18/18/
    jennifer-aniston-diet-workout-body
webmd.com/fitness-exercise/features/
    the-top-6-exercise-excuses-and-how-to-beat-them
brainhq.com/brain-resources/everyday-brain-fitness/physical-exercise
cooperaerobics.com/Health-Tips/Stress-Less/Research-on-the-Benefits-
    of-Exercise-and-Mental-He.aspx
helpguide.org/articles/healthy-living/the-mental-health-benefits-of-
    exercise.htm
cobbcsb.com/the-mental-health-benefits-of-exercise/
Sandoui, Ana. "How Can Exercise Improve Body Image?"
    medicalnewstoday.com/articles/317958.php

"I Aspire to Look and Feel Healthy Like the Posts Convey." ncbi.nlm. nih.gov/pmc/articles/PMC6086030/

popsugar.com/fitness/Jennifer-Lawrence-Diet-Exercise-35480083

"The Connection between Heart Health and Brain Health." cooperinstitute.org/pub/news.cfm?id=182

cooperaerobics.com/Health-Tips/Fitness-Files/The-Aerobic-Strength-Balance.aspx

health.harvard.edu/staying-healthy/the-ideal-stretching-routine

cooperinstitute.org/fitnessgram

Chapter 5

psychologytoday.com/us/blog/shame/201305/the-difference-between-guilt-and-shame

Burney, J. and H. J. Irwin. "Shame and Guilt in Women with Eating-Disorder Symptomatology." ncbi.nlm.nih.gov/pubmed/10661368

webmd.com/diet/features/emotional-eating-feeding-feelings#1

health.harvard.edu/blog/why-eating-slowly-may-help-you-feel-full-faster-20101019605

livestrong.com/article/480254-how-long-does-it-take-your-brain-to-register-that-the-stomach-is-full/

huffpost.com/entry/calorie-count-searches-2016-google_n_585bf03de4b0eb5864855af5

cooperinstitute.org/2017/09/05/dietary-carbohydrate-facts-and-misconceptions-15772

webmd.com/diet/guide/vitamin-d-deficiency

nof.org/news/54-million-americans-affected-by-osteoporosis-and-low-bone-mass/

hsph.harvard.edu/nutritionsource/what-should-you-eat/protein/

self.com/story/9-high-fat-foods-actually-good-for-you

foodrevolution.org/blog/eating-the-rainbow-health-benefits/

hsph.harvard.edu/nutritionsource/what-should-you-eat/vegetables-and-fruits/

amazon.com/Cooper-Clinic-Solution-Diet-Revolution/dp/0963596926

Chapter 6

harpersbazaar.com/celebrity/red-carpet-dresses/a13999611/
meghan-markle-carolyn-bessette-kennedy-outfit/

amazon.com/Instyle-New-Secrets-Style-Complete/dp/1603200827

glamour.com/story/jessica-alba-pregnancy-body-image

Chapter 7

blog.siriusxm.com/adele-celebrates-new-album-25-with-intimate-
listener-qa-on-the-spectrum/

usatoday.com/story/life/people/2014/05/01/
emma-stone-body-image-spider-man/8541525/

Juvonen, J.and S. Graham, S. "Bullying in Schools: The
Power of Bullies and the Plight of Victims." *Annual Review
of Psychology.* Annual Reviews. **65**: 159–85. doi:10.1146/
annurev-psych-010213-115030. PMID 23937767

allure.com/gallery/celebrities-body-shamed

Chapter 8

facebook.com/amightygirl/posts/as-a-child-i-never-heard-one-
woman-say-to-me-i-love-my-body-not-my-mother-my-
eld/891714234198224/

cnn.com/2015/11/03/health/teens-tweens-media-screen-use-report/
index.html

verywellfamily.com/media-and-teens-body-image-2611245

thebodypositive.org

cbsnews.com/news/susan-boyle-announces-she-has-aspergers-more-on-
the-developmental-disorder/

Susan Walker, M.S., L.P.C.

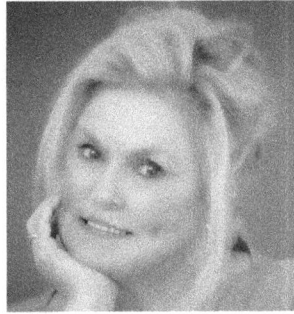

Susan Walker, MS, LPC, is a psychotherapist and the clinical director for Walker Wellness Clinic at Cooper Aerobics Center. She and her husband, Philip Walker, MS, CEO, have clinics in Dallas and Houston that specialize in body image, eating disorders, depression, anxiety, and stress. Susan is dedicated to empowering women and men by helping them enhance their body image via techniques she has developed over her years of clinical practice. She has been active in the Women's Council of Dallas and the Dallas Symphony Orchestra League. Susan has also served on the advisory board at the Cooper Institute for Childhood Obesity Prevention.

Susan lives in Dallas, Texas, with her husband Philip and a lovely but mischievous Siamese cat named Biggles.

www.ingramcontent.com/pod-product-compliance
Lightning Source LLC
Chambersburg PA
CBHW062053270326
41931CB00013B/3061